Living the
Good Life

Living the Good Life

*Health and Success
for You—for Canada*

Revised and Updated Edition

DAVID PATCHELL-EVANS

ECW PRESS

Copyright © 2015, 2012, 2011, 2002, 2000 David Patchell-Evans
Published by ECW Press
665 Gerrard Street East, Toronto, Ontario M4M 1Y2
416-694-3348 / info@ecwpress.com

LIBRARY AND ARCHIVES CANADA CATALOGUING IN PUBLICATION
Patchell-Evans, David, author
Living the good life : health and success for you—for Canada /
David Patchell-Evans.

ISBN 978-1-77041-302-3 (pbk.), 978-1-77090-824-6 (pdf), 978-1-77090-825-3 (epub)

1. Patchell-Evans, David. 2. Exercise. 3. Physical fitness. 4. Health. I. Title.

RA776.P373 2015   613.7   C2015-903134-6

Front cover photo: Beth Hayhurst
Back cover: Canada flag image © iStock
Interior design: Troy Cunningham
Printing: Friesens   25   24   23   22

PRINTED AND BOUND IN CANADA

To Kilee and Tygre, my two precious daughters,
who enlighten and enrich my life beyond measure.

To my beautiful wife and soulmate, Silken,
and to William and Kate, my new stepson and stepdaughter:
you make our home and happiness complete.

To my brothers, Ed and Jerry, for always being there.

To Jane, my indispensable second-in-charge
for almost four decades,
and who I consider to be a sister by rites of passage.

And to the lady who started it all,
my mom, Dorothy, now 95 and going strong.
Thanks for everything!

CONTENTS

PREFACE

I wrote this book because I want to encourage you to live the good life. What is the good life? It's about health. It's about feeling at home in your body. It's about allowing your body to become the best it can be. It's the feeling of energy and alertness you feel when you're in good shape. It's about the confidence with which you meet life challenges. It's knowing that you can achieve far more than you ever dreamed. It's the sense of yourself as a body, mind, heart, and soul—a whole being, vibrant and alive.

Contrary to what we're told by media and even fitness "gurus," being healthy and fit is not difficult. It's easy. I hope I can convince you in these pages just how easy it is. When you experience how easy it is, you'll also experience how joyful and life affirming it is to feel your health improve and the mastery of your life increase.

Writing this book has been a journey—a journey of putting down on paper the thoughts and feelings I've carried about fitness for a long time, the thoughts and feelings that drive the success of GoodLife Fitness and my own life.

I am grateful for all the wonderful GoodLife staff at our clubs and in our home office, whose dedication to caring for and about our members makes GoodLife one of the top fitness club chains in the world. I also want to thank all of our GoodLife members, especially those who share their personal stories in this book. The stories have touched my heart, as they affirm so many of the positive things that can happen in people's lives when they take control of their health and fitness. Without all of you club members, GoodLife would not exist. So to you, the members of GoodLife—over one million strong and growing—I say: YOU are the reason I wrote this book.

DAVID PATCHELL-EVANS

WILD TOES, DUDE!

There I was, walking on a beautiful beach in Hawaii. The sand was hot and soft at the same time. The cooling trade winds, the clear blue water matching the sky—it was a perfect day of no cares and complete relaxation. It was magic.

Set back slightly from the beach was an area being claimed by mangrove swamps, a combination of plants and brush tough enough to resist the assaults of salt, tides, moisture, and temperature swings. Looking rather out of place, a man was reclining on one of those plastic folding chairs. His body was covered with tattoos, not as common a sight 15 years ago as today. He was deep in concentration, making a necklace out of small, delicate seashells. With his long and unkempt hair, he looked like a biker, but a biker with an artistic side. I called out a friendly "hey" to him. He looked me up and down, and his mouth curled into an amused smile. Then he gestured toward my feet and said, "Wild toes, dude!"

No big surprise there, if you've ever seen my feet.

I have rheumatoid arthritis, which has taken its toll on the shape of my toes. If you've ever been swimming with me or seen me in flip-flops, you may have seen my twisted toes, kind of like pretzels gone wild. My big toes touch my baby toes. The other toes pile on top. I have big two-inch bunions. I told my kids they are magic toes. However, I knew from this man's jovial tone that he wasn't making fun of me. He was just stating a fact, no offence meant—or taken. I approached him, and we struck up a conversation.

Interesting guy. It turned out he had been a pro surfer and now made his living as a Harley-Davidson mechanic. He also said he liked to spend his spare time picking up small seashells and stringing them together with beads to make bracelets, which he sold to five jewelry stores. I thought the bracelets looked really cool and bought some as gifts for my daughters.

Mr. Tattooed Harley-Davidson Biker Surfer Guy asked me, the Wild Toes Dude, if I wanted a drink. Taking some long pulls on our cold beers, we sat back and exchanged stories.

A couple of days later, I decided to go surfing for the day, so I needed to rent a surfboard. I wanted a big, soft, easier-to-control board, since it was my first time surfing in bigger waves. I couldn't find what I needed in the regular rental place. However, across the street was a small dress shop. All around the dress shop were surfboards. Seemed a little weird! I found an open-air rental shack near it. Despite its size, there was a great collection of over 30 colourful boards, all propped up at the back. A rather intimidating woman wrapped in an astounding, colourful muumuu came to the counter. I asked about the surfboards, and she began yelling for her husband to come out and help me. He didn't answer. So she yelled louder. Still no response. She yelled some more. All the while, he was standing right behind her. I didn't know whether to play along or point him out to her. A wide grin showed he was clearly enjoying himself. Luckily, the decision was taken from me. He leaned forward, probably sensing he had gone far enough, and said, "Yes, dear?" into her ear. She was not impressed with his antics, but he survived to live another day in paradise.

I don't remember his name, but he was a classic Jimmy Buffett type of guy. I like Jimmy Buffett a lot. He is known as the king of tropical paradise, and here I was standing barefoot in paradise, so I had a good feeling about the guy. He was mid-60s, fit, and seemed just kinda happy. Turns out he was the one who made all the surfboards standing at the back of the shop.

"So you need a surfboard," he said. Just like the tattooed guy, he looked me up and down. His eyes locked onto my feet. "Wild toes, dude!" he said.

Two different guys, the exact same words. Yes, I guess my toes really are wild looking (anyway, I appreciated the word "wild" instead of "weird"). He helped me choose a surfboard and then set about waxing it for me. I kept asking him how much the rental cost would be, and he replied, "Oh, I'll figure that out when you get back . . . no hurry."

"Where should I surf?" I asked.

"I don't know right now," he said. "Wait—just give me a minute. The answer will come."

I thought, well, what am I doing with this board if the surf shop guy doesn't know where I can find the right waves? Hmm . . .

Right then, the phone rang. He picked it up and replied to the caller. "How high's the surf? Where is that, you say? Great! Thanks for calling."

He proceeded to give me detailed instructions on where to go to find the good waves—not the biggest waves, but waves I could handle with my "wild toes."

"Wait a minute . . . you just said you didn't know."

He grinned. "I put it out there, man. You know, your question . . . I asked the universe. Telepathy or something like that, and a friend heard me and called in the info you need. Works every time."

I went to the spot he suggested, and he was totally right. The waves were fantastic and just right for me. All the others surfing at that spot were locals, so I realized he had sent me to a great spot that only the locals really knew about. That was a good feeling. It made feel at home.

When I returned the board, I asked him to recommend a good restaurant.

"OK, no problem, dude, just go down the street," he said, chuckling. "Park at the old folks' home. Walk around to the front beachside. It's locals only, and it has great steak. Just send two Millers in to the cook in the kitchen, and he will give you the best steak on this entire island."

Wow! I'll say! It was the best steak, and I had just had the best day. I often think back on those two men and how they both remarked on my toes, and remember the spirit of friendship I felt and the island magic.

However, it could have been otherwise. I could have chosen to get upset at their teasing. I could have chosen to feel awkward and uncomfortable. I could have chosen to see them as saying something insensitive, because, after all, we're not supposed to say inappropriate things about people's physical appearance. That was not the choice I made.

Why? Because over the years I've reached a level of self-acceptance. I have made the decision to focus on what's good, on what's right, not wrong. To not let negative thoughts get in the way of all the good ones. To focus on what I can do physically, not what I can't. To be in the moment, being present to the gifts life gives to me. I was once an elite athlete, a champion rower, and believe me, it was hard at the age of 32 to be diagnosed with rheumatoid arthritis and to be in so much pain I couldn't even turn a doorknob. Sure my joints are affected. By the time of that surfing day in Hawaii, I was in my 50s and had learned that it doesn't matter if I'm imperfect, if my body no longer looks like it did when I was a competitive rower headed for the Olympics. Even though I'm the owner of a large chain of fitness clubs, I don't have to look perfect. Just do my best.

After years of watching people in my fitness clubs doing their workouts to develop the best level of health for themselves, I saw that almost nobody has a perfect body. Even people with what the rest of us would call a perfect body find fault with themselves. I also saw that all those imperfect bodies seemed to exude a sense of comfort and flexibility, brought on by the good feelings that come from exercise. In short, I frequently saw club members getting happier with themselves despite not being perfect. Their attitude rubbed off on me because I, too, came to accept my own sometimes less than cooperative arthritic body. I realized that in fact I was very blessed. I have a business I love. I have a wonderful family. I have great friends. I have a full life. It didn't matter that I had wild toes. In fact, my toes make me distinguished! Or so I tell all my friends.

What I have learned is that there is a great power in self-acceptance—that if you accept who, what, and where you are each and every day, in that moment you will sense an even stronger underlying feeling—and that feeling is happiness.

This book is about living a good life. It's about making peace with yourself and then bringing all the energy and vitality you can to living each day. It's about releasing judgment. Don't judge yourself or others. It's about connecting with the world beyond your door. It's about the freedom to be. It's about awareness. It's about walking on the earth with a spring in your step. It's about laughter and humour. It's about giving and receiving. It's about moving around—about getting off the couch and into your body's desire to move. It's about feeling grounded in your body. It's about allowing yourself to discover the happiness that's right there inside you right now waiting to be found.

You can't find happiness if you're judging yourself or selling yourself short. On that surfing holiday in Hawaii, I saw the meeting with the two men as a time of making human connection. Because we made this connection, I ended up with some great bracelets to give to friends and family, an awesome surfboard, an even more awesome place to surf, and a great dinner from a cook who enjoyed his two Millers in his kitchen. What could have been more fulfilling than that day? You see, when you carry happiness inside, your brain will interpret events in a more positive way. It will show you where the opportunities are to have something wonderful happen.

Just because you're imperfect (and who isn't?) doesn't lessen your ability to live comfortably in your own skin. There is a Buddhist teacher who often talks about what he calls the spirit of welcoming. Happiness happens, he says, when we welcome every day into our lives. "The first person you have to welcome each day when you wake up from sleep is yourself. Welcome yourself into life, and you will be happy."

So let me welcome you to this book where we'll be exploring all kinds of thoughts, feelings, musings, insights, questions, hopes, and dreams about what a healthy and good life is and can be. Find the part of yourself that's wild. For me, it's my toes. For you, maybe it's your hair, or your ears, or your long legs, or that dimple in your cheek, or your propensity to like crazy clothes, or your unique laugh.

You know, the words both of those men spoke to me that day have turned out to be healing words. Every time I feel a bit down, or when I'm stressed, or things aren't going the way I want them to, I hear them say, "Wild toes, dude!"—and then I smile.

CHAPTER ONE

THE SIMPLICITY OF BEING FIT

WHY IS IT that less than 20 percent of the population exercises regularly? Why does the other 80 percent not bother? Why are they mainly sedentary, or think physical activity is taking out the garbage once every week? Because they think fitness is hard. They think they can't do it, or that they don't have time to do it.

I'm here to tell you that it's easy and that you can do it. The whole point of this book is to help you see how simple it is to be fit—and what you will gain in your life as a result.

I'm not a fitness guru. I'm not going to tell you about the latest fad diets or give you detailed descriptions of complicated exercises and fitness equipment. I'm going to tell you some of what I've learned in my 36 years in the fitness industry. I'm a person who cares very much about well-being and health. I want to see a society in which greater numbers of people achieve total well-being. I want to see people make decisions for health and vitality. I want to play a part in helping them put those decisions into action. This is the driving vision of my entire professional life.

This passion for health and fitness—and the knowledge that it's simple—has led my company, GoodLife Fitness, to become the largest chain of fitness clubs in Canada and one of the largest in the world. We have 350 clubs, over 13,000 staff, and more than one million members. We have only one reason for being: to make you fit and healthy, to make you believe you can do this, to get you off the couch and into your own body. In fact, throughout this book, you'll be reading some exciting comments from people from across Canada who have done just that and have really gotten into the good life.

MY OWN JOURNEY
INTO FITNESS

MY OWN LEVEL of activity as a child was not all that unusual. I didn't spend my childhood as an athlete in training. In the High Park area of Toronto, where I grew up, I was just a regular active kid. I played hockey, went to summer camps, and spent time at the family cottage until about age 12, when I became old enough to begin summer jobs. I seemed to always have jobs that required physical labour. I rode a bicycle to make deliveries for a drugstore. I worked at a gas station—I used to make a game of how fast I could run from one car to another to pump the gas, jumping between the pumps and swinging on them. I didn't realize that bicycling and my gas station antics amounted to aerobic training. The High Park area is really hilly, and biking up and down those slopes from 4:00 p.m. to 8:00 p.m. every day got my legs into great shape. When I became a teenager, hockey became football and karate.

A little later, when I became interested in rowing and was trying out for the national team, my bicycling experience served me well. The team recruiters used to test prospective rowers on a bicycle, and I was one of the best. That summer of drugstore deliveries helped open the door for me to become a Canadian champion rower later on.

You might think doing such physical jobs would put the idea of "fitness" into my head, but it didn't. It wasn't until I was in a physical rehab clinic, totally torn apart, that I began to understand what the body needs to be healthy. At age 19, during the second week of my first year at the University of Western Ontario (now Western University), I had a devastating motorcycle accident. A car cut me off, and the motorcycle I was riding fell on top of me. In one of those bursts of strength you get when you're in an emergency and your nerves are all fired up, I threw the motorcycle off me. I couldn't move for several hours after that.

My clavicle was broken. My shoulder was paralyzed, dislocated, the tendons and chest muscles torn. I was a total mess. In fact, my right side and arm were about four inches lower. I ended up going for rehabilitation to Western University's renowned Fowler Kennedy Clinic, my first introduction to the clinic's founder, Dr. Peter Fowler.

While I was at the clinic, I watched people in all stages of rehabilitation, some recovering from accidents far more severe than mine. I became acutely aware of the fragility of life, how limited and finite it is—and not just life, but quality of life. To me, these two things are similar, but also very different. One is about staying alive. If you've had a stroke or a heart attack, or if you've been in a car accident, you're happy just to be alive. You say to yourself, "Thank God, I'm still here." But then you get to rehab and the question becomes, "What's the quality of my life going to be?"

There I was, about to turn 20, and I had to ask myself, "Am I going to have one shoulder four inches lower than the other, or am I going to get into shape and build it back up?"

In the clinic I was surrounded by people all going through the trauma of some kind of injury. At the same time, the top athletes at the university were there to use the equipment because it was so much more advanced than anything else available at the time. So, right beside me, really motivated athletes were working out. There were also athletes who had been injured, and they were the most motivated of all.

I took all this in and thought about it at length. As a young university student, I was also at the stage of pondering, "What am I going to do with my life? What career do I want?" At the clinic I saw the satisfaction that arises from looking after others, from helping make sure they have a decent quality of life, even in the face of accidents and injuries.

For the rest of that school year, I did rehab and tried to get back into shape. At first I did 20 minutes three times per week. (The insurance company had said I would get funding for being disabled.) So I said to the physiotherapist, "What would happen if I came more often?" He looked at me like the answer was just obvious. "Well," he said, "you have a better chance of healing and a more complete recovery." So following the athletes' examples, I went in daily for 30 minutes, then daily for two hours, progressing to twice a day for two hours. Seven months later, the school term ended. I realized that I was no longer disabled. That started my career.

That summer I first got a job as a lumberjack and then later as a lifeguard. In the fall I took up rowing to build up my right arm. I had come to Western to go to its business school. I had also taken a physical education course, which at first I didn't treat all that seriously. However, it turned out to be really interesting, and in my second year I took another one. This one was instrumental in forming my ideas about the direction I wanted to go. The professors kept touching on the benefits to your head and your heart that come from doing physical activity. I ended up switching from the business school to physical education.

During my third year I rowed competitively and took a course on the philosophy of physical education given by Jack Fairs. Jack kept talking about how, through most of history, people have thought of the body as one thing, the mind as another, and the soul as still another. His point was that they're really the same thing, and he gave example after example. I thought he was a great professor, despite the fact that I sometimes fell asleep in his class because I had been out snowplowing the night before. That was another hat I wore in university: I started a snowplowing business that paid my way through school but also, more importantly, gave me a credit rating.

I also took business courses. One was an exploration of what kind of business I would like to establish. I did my business plan on how to open a squash club. I had come to realize that I wanted to do something in the recreation/fitness field. I wanted to make a difference for people using my skills—to be the initiator of a fitness-related business that would create opportunities for people to lead healthy lives and to benefit the way I had.

Often what you learn in business courses doesn't prepare you to be your own boss. You learn skills that enable you to work for someone else who has a vision. The people who own companies are the ones with vision. They hire people with business degrees to help run their companies. I wanted both the vision and the ability to run my own company.

It occurred to me that there was nobody out there with a vision about fitness who knew anything about business. So I decided to put the two together—I had the physical education training and the business training, so next I worked hard at developing salesmanship. Additionally, I took courses such as exercise physiology, scientific training techniques, a variety of practical sports applications, and so forth—things that would enable me to run a club. I knew how to make the body go fast, and I understood a balance sheet.

By December of 1977, after graduating with an honours degree in physical education, I was taking my first year of the master's degree in exercise physiology. However, it snowed like crazy that winter. I had built up my snowplowing business and plowed every single night for three weeks, sleeping only every second day for three or four hours. I made a lot of money, but I fell asleep during two of my exams. The professors thought I had my priorities all wrong—that I was more focused on making money than my studies. In March, they told me to take the year off to think. I took the summer off and kept rowing and training for the national team. I got my snowplowing business organized for another winter. I had some fun along the way and trained and raced hard.

By 1980, I had won five Canadian rowing championships (two in 1977, two in 1979, and one in 1980).

The year before the 1980 Olympic Games, as part of our training for the tryouts, the national rowing team said we needed to work out on Nautilus equipment. Till then I had been lifting free weights. I was familiar with the Nautilus equipment from my time spent in rehab for my injured shoulders. I found a fitness club that had the equipment.

Every day while I was working out, I asked the owner questions about his business.

One day he said to me, "If you're so interested in this club, why don't you buy it? It's for sale."

"Why is it for sale?" I asked.

He simply said, "I'm going broke."

"No problem," I said. "I'll come back at nine o'clock after rowing practice, and we'll talk about it."

I came back at the appointed hour with a 12-pack of beer, and by midnight we had made a deal. When the club opened the next morning, I opened it as the owner.

That was in 1979. The money I had made the previous year in those big snowfalls gave me enough capital to get started. The club was called Canada Pro Fitness, located at Adelaide and Cheapside Streets in London, Ontario. That was my first club, the forerunner of the GoodLife Fitness chain.

My snowplowing business had grown considerably. I had five trucks, about a dozen employees, and 120 lots to plow every time it snowed—I made good money. I was also a carded athlete, receiving some government funding for my training, and I had a paid teaching assistantship as part of my master's program.

In doing the business plan for my first club, I discovered that no one in fitness clubs knew anything about fitness. Their focus was on sales. They were business people. And at the universities, where all the physical education specialists were, no one knew anything about sales. The opportunity presented to me was to bring these two worlds together— to learn more about business (particularly sales), and about fitness, and apply it all to my passion for making people better. I had reached a high level of fitness through my rowing and my physical education courses and had experienced physical recovery in rehab. I had a good idea of what was necessary to achieve a high quality of life in terms of exercise and fitness. Most importantly, I had a dream that this was what I would do. I would help people get the most out of their body, mind, and soul. I would introduce them to the good life. I just didn't know I would call it that yet.

IT MAKES
PERFECT SENSE

YOU DECIDE HOW fit you're going to be. This was the core philosophy of GoodLife right from that very first club: to give you the control and the means to achieve a healthy body and a sharp mind. You can make a conscious decision about how well you want to be, and that decision will affect your entire quality of life.

Six months after my injury, I worked as a lumberjack, then as a lifeguard. Ten months after the accident, I was part of a competitive rowing team. Those were my choices. Not everyone has to pursue a sport. That was just my particular spin on things. I'll come back to the differences between athletics and fitness later in this book.

It was in the 1990s that medical associations in the United States and Canada began saying that fitness actually increases the length of your life. I knew from my own experience that fitness made people better. I knew it made them happier. I knew it gave them more energy, made them more optimistic, and improved their self-esteem. It just made sense that fitness would also help people live longer. We all know that if we treat a car well and keep it well maintained, it will last longer. Yet we don't seem to understand that about our own bodies. We've known for hundreds of years that how well you treat a horse determines how well the horse rides. If you had a horse worth $100,000, you'd give it the best food, make sure it got good exercise, and look after its health. Most people don't do that for themselves. Most people don't think they're worth as much as a $100,000 horse.

When I opened my first fitness club, it made sense to me to take advantage of this opportunity. Although fitness clubs had existed for a while, they were called "health spas," and the emphasis was on passivity and relaxation. There's nothing wrong with relaxation, but the other side of the equation is activity. Just as you don't get to enjoy your paycheque until you've worked, so, with fitness, you have to put in a little effort before you get to the "relax and enjoy" part.

The really neat thing about fitness is you don't have to spend a lot of time to get unbelievable benefits. You do have to continue with it—it can't be just a "sometime" thing. We have to eat all the time; we have to bathe all the time. Fitness doesn't take any more time than preparing a meal or taking a bath. If you spend half an hour three times a week doing fitness activities, you'll be in better shape than 90 percent of the population.

Another advantage I had from my training background was that I realized there are options other than just lifting barbells. There is more than one way to shape up your heart and lungs. There is more than one way to build up your muscles. Now science and technology have made it even easier, because we've got exercise equipment today that didn't exist before. If you can get to the point where you are exercising three times a week for six months—whether by using equipment or by other means—you will know and understand the benefits of fitness, because you'll feel these benefits. You'll feel them in your body and you'll feel them in your spirit. And you'll keep on doing it.

TURNING POINT

I DON'T WANT to imply that if you take the road to fitness you will never have any rough times. Life can hit us broadside with things we don't expect. It's a matter of deciding that no matter what happens, you will be the best you can be. The accident I had when I was 19 was a turning point in my life: if I hadn't gone through rehab and been turned on to fitness, I probably would just have gone into the business world.

However, another even more dramatic turning point happened when I was 32.

I had been competing in the World Rowing Masters championships, and I had won three medals. Yet when I woke up the next morning, I found I couldn't get out of bed. I was in unbelievable pain. Every joint in my body hurt. I couldn't carry my gym bag, I couldn't open the door, I couldn't turn the key in the car ignition. I had to walk on the sides of my feet because they hurt so bad. I couldn't put my elbows on the table because they had grown by two inches, full of lumpy mush. I had bumps all over my body. At work someone had to help me lift the lightest weight. I couldn't turn the bicycle wheels. I owned about seven or eight clubs at the time, all of which demanded my attention, and I felt like I was falling apart because of the tremendous pain. I also couldn't sleep.

No one could diagnose the problem at first. I tried massage and chiropractic, but nothing helped. About two months after this nightmare began, my mother became ill, and I took her to the hospital. The doctor on call was Duncan McKinley, who had been a friend of mine at university and had played in the Canadian Football League. We needed to adjust my mother's position on the bed to make her more comfortable. Duncan asked me to help, but I fumbled, unable to lift my mother.

"What's wrong?" he asked.

"I can't use my hands," I said.

He looked at my hands and then back at me and replied, "Well, Patch, you've got arthritis."

No one had picked up on this, because you don't expect "Mr. Fitness Guy" to have arthritis. Duncan sent me to some specialists for tests, and they found the RA factor in my blood—I had rheumatoid arthritis.

The first thing they told me was not to exercise. I paid attention to that advice for about a month, but the only thing that happened was I got weaker. I had weighed about 210 pounds on a six-foot-five frame and was pretty strong, and my weight dropped to 180 pounds just from muscle wasting away. So I disobeyed doctors' orders and started to exercise. At first I had to get someone to help me just move at all: a form of personal training in its infancy. Gradually I got to the point where I could turn the bicycle wheel by myself and work through the pain. When I did that, I felt better afterwards. The doctors tried different drugs on me. I learned all about arthritis attacks and how they come in cycles. I experimented with nutrition and worked my way right through the medical library looking up information on my condition. What I found was that mental attitude makes a huge difference. The same skills you need as a business person to be successful and you need as an athlete to excel, you must apply to healing your body. My illness, and my efforts to cope with it and break through it, taught me the most important lesson about fitness and about running a fitness-oriented business.

The big door that opened for me was a far greater understanding about not taking things for granted. When I was having constant pain with every motion, I no longer took movement for granted. This pushed me to a whole new level in terms of my humanity and empathy. Now I understand when a 79-year-old person comes into one of my clubs and says, "I can't do stuff." Or when someone comes in after having surgery and says, "I'm having trouble recuperating." Or when a person says, "I've weighed 40 pounds too much for a long time, and I just can't seem to lose it." I have an idea of how hard it is.

Very few people in the fitness industry really understand what it's like to be old or weakened. But I became "old" at 32, and I had to work to recover the quality of life I valued. This has made an enormous difference in how I run my clubs and how I have designed my business to take care of people's needs.

"BE THE BEST
YOU CAN BE"

THE EMPHASIS IN fitness, as I see it, is this: to train people for success—their success. The purpose is not to make judgments, but to help each person become the best he or she can be. I know this is a cliché bandied about by motivational speakers and in self-help books—"Be the best you can be"—but the fact that it's overworked doesn't make it less true.

To me, being the best you can be means becoming as highly functional as possible, and not just physically. Exercise makes you smarter—you're getting more oxygen to the brain. Studies show that children who exercise at school get better marks. It's not a big jump to say that working people who exercise get better money. Studies show that physically active people are more productive, have far fewer absences from work, and make at least 20 percent more on average.

If you know that fitness makes you feel better—makes you be better—then it can encourage you not to accept mediocrity in yourself, and that will have positive effects in many areas of your life. You will reach the "better" only when you push the basics. You will know what it's like to be good at something, to achieve your own personal best—not compared to anyone else—only if you push your own limits. Your limits are just things you're used to.

Feeling better in my mid-40s, I went climbing by myself once when visiting Palm Springs. I had noticed some small mountains nearby. I hadn't done any real climbing since I got arthritis, but they didn't look that high. I left the hotel at 5:30 a.m. and began the climb. It was really steep, and before long I was clambering over rocks and boulders, wondering what on earth I was trying to prove—it was like being on nature's StairMaster. As the sun rose behind me, I saw a sudden glint higher up. A coyote was looking down at me from 75 feet above. The sunlight had caught the edge of the cliff, making the coyote's fur shine golden. He thought he was hidden. It was the most beautiful sight, and I would never have seen it if I hadn't pushed myself to try that climb. On my way back down I saw several more coyotes, watching me from a distance.

I was back for breakfast at 9:00 a.m. Do you think the other hotel guests had any clue what I had just enjoyed? It couldn't have happened if I hadn't had a good fitness level, developed through exercising six times a week, half an hour a day, for the previous 10 years. It doesn't even have to be six times a week. You can exercise three times a week and still be amazingly fit. Two days after I saw the coyotes, I climbed up by the gondola in Palm Springs for my very first overhang—scary, challenging, and rewarding. I can still remember that feeling of accomplishment.

It's all about gaining a sense of control over yourself. I won't say control over your life, because many things happen to us in life that we can't control. However, you can have control of yourself and how you respond to those things. When people first come into a fitness club, many have never exercised. They've never participated in any kind of physical activity. Fitness gives you control. Your body will degenerate if you don't use it, so use it! Everyone ages, but if you're fit you're going to age a lot more slowly.

A lot of self-help methods are based on mental discipline, or on working through emotional issues so you see them in a new light, or on doing spiritual work such as learning forgiveness and compassion. What these approaches lack is that they don't get the body into the equation. The health of your body influences what you experience in your mind. There is no split. If you can engage your whole spirit in the pursuit of fitness—not just your intellect, not just your emotions—you'll discover what it is to be a whole person.

Your body needs and wants exercise. It needs it every 48 hours just to recover from the stresses of everyday life. It needs it to maintain strong bones. It needs it to have a lower heart rate, so you don't have fatty acids in your arteries. Your head needs exercise, too. If you burn off stress, you think more clearly. All these things allow your soul to be free, because you feel "in sync."

BEST DOESN'T
MEAN PERFECT

ONE THING I think is really important in the field of fitness is that it's not about perfection. Being your best, in terms of fitness, is not about being perfect. We all know people who go overboard, who seem totally addicted to exercise, going at it for hours every day. But such obsessive exercisers are few in the overall population. There are a lot fewer compulsive exercisers than there are compulsive overeaters. There are a lot fewer compulsive exercisers than there are compulsive workers, compulsive worriers, or compulsive TV watchers.

At GoodLife I have a saying: "Good enough is good enough." What we try to do is help establish a person's objectives. You might say, for example, "I want to lose 10 pounds, have a resting heart rate of 60 beats per minute, and be able to play with my kids without getting tired out." You establish these things as goals and decide on a time frame in which to get them done.

When you've reached your goals, you have three choices. First, you can pat yourself on the back, go home, and do nothing further, which means that in the same time it took to get you into shape you'll also get out of shape again. A lot of people think fitness is something you achieve and then it just stays there. That's not true.

The second choice is to say, "Good enough is good enough," and then maintain the gains. You've reached your goals and you have enough energy. All you have to do is show up three times a week to exercise, and you'll keep your level of fitness. For example, if you do 20 minutes on the stair machine and eight strength exercises that work the whole body three times a week, that's all you'll have to do forever. That's phenomenally easy.

The hard part is the first six months—but anyone can do six months, when you really think about it. This psychology is foreign to our culture. Most people think, "As soon as I've got to here, I've got to get to there." You don't have to. We know if you do two good strength workouts a week, it will help you get stronger. If you do three cardiovascular workouts a week, you'll keep your heart and lungs in good shape.

The third choice is the constant struggle to be better, to keep pushing. If I can walk 100 feet, then I can go 1,000 feet, then 10,000 feet. Then I have to run 1,000 feet, then 10,000 feet. That's well and good if you want to do that. However, you don't have to. All you have to do is work to get the optimum level of fitness for you and then maintain it. You don't have to keep pushing unless you want to.

Let's say you get into a fitness routine and you work out on several pieces of equipment. You move 20 pounds for two weeks. Then you decide to try 22 pounds. My job as a fitness professional might be to tell you that, for you, 22 is fine. You might think, "I've run three miles. Now I have to run 10." You don't. Anything you run after three miles would be for your own satisfaction; it's not because you need it for your fitness. The physiological difference between two hours of running and just half an hour is between 2 and 5 percent. Do you burn more fat? Yes. Does your heart get more efficient? Yes—but only marginally. You don't have to become an exercise fanatic to enjoy the phenomenal benefits that fitness will give you.

Another issue affecting your ability to be your best is time. People often say, "I don't have time to exercise." Yet numerous studies have shown that, at a minimum, you are 20 percent more productive if you exercise. If you're 20 percent more productive, that means you create 33 more hours per week by exercising. Where do the 33 hours come from? You get them because your decisions are 20 percent faster, you have 20 percent less anxiety, your sleep is 20 percent deeper. You create time by exercising. If you exercise for half an hour three times a week, you gain the equivalent of 33 hours a week in terms of productivity. You give up an hour and a half to gain 33.

By avoiding fitness, you're not saving any time. You're actually losing it. Invariably, people who are leaders in business, politics, sports, and life in general are physically active.

WE ARE
PHYSICAL BEINGS

FITNESS CENTRES YOU. Fitness underscores the reality that you are a physical being. It wasn't all that long ago that we were hunters and gatherers and our survival depended on our ability to move and be flexible and strong. You are built for physical activity. If you don't do it, you can create disease. When you don't participate in activity, you're working counter to your body, which means you're lowering the quality of every other aspect of your life.

In these times of rapid technological change, which hasn't even begun to peak yet, people often feel out of control, powerless to stop change or to navigate through it. Stress is epidemic in our society.

The things you definitely can control are your attitude and your body. You decide if you're going to be happy. You decide if you're going to be fit. Get rid of all the absolutes. I don't know of many people who think they have perfect bodies.

When I give my introductory seminar to all new staff, typically several thousand a year (broken into group seminars regionally across Canada), I always ask which of them has a perfect body. Few are bold enough to stick their hands up. The question has to be, "Who is happy with their body?"

Still, most people wouldn't put their hands up on that one, either, because most people think their body has to be better. People who appear to be in great shape aren't always happy with their bodies, either. We have to get away from this need for perfection to "it's right for me."

IT ALL
COMES TOGETHER

THE ACCIDENT I had when I was in university made me aware that there are "roses," things in life to be enjoyed. Life had to be more than just survival. There had to be quality of life. Yet it wasn't until I got sick with rheumatoid arthritis that I really figured out the concept of the "soul" in fitness. It wasn't until every move hurt that I understood my body's role in nurturing my spirit. The best thing that ever happened to me was getting arthritis. It awakened me to how good every single moment is. It made me realize that caring for my body, giving it the activity it needs—even when the pain is so great I think, "No way am I doing this"—is the very best thing I can do for myself.

Making a commitment to look after your body's need for physical activity brings balance to the soul, the intellect, the heart, and the body. It puts it all together. At some deep, basic level we all know this. We know it, but most of us don't do anything about it.

How we get from knowing to doing is what the rest of this book is about. Knowing that something is good for you is not enough to make you do it. You have to feel good doing it. Along the way we'll share some experiences of people who have gone from knowing to doing, stories of ordinary people, not athletic superstars, who came to GoodLife Fitness looking for a way to enhance their health and well-being and made amazing gains.

CHAPTER TWO

THE SIMPLICITY
OF BEING HAPPY

IT'S SAID THAT the Inuit people of the North have over a hundred words for "snow." Each word has a slightly different nuance; for example, one might mean "ice-covered snow" and another "slushy snow." Whichever word was chosen for "snow," the listener would know exactly what the speaker meant. In the English language, we can have the opposite problem. We often use one word that can mean many different things. Like "love." If you say, "I love you," do you mean you are in love with the person romantically? That you love him or her as a good friend? That you love him or her as a parent or sibling? That you love how the person is behaving? (Maybe he or she is being really witty today and you say, "I love you when you're like that!") Depending on the context, you could mean any one of those interpretations of the word "love."

"Happiness" is another such word. We all agree that we want to be happy. In reality, we all have different ideas about what that would look like for us in our lives and different ways of describing it. Happiness is very important to us. We believe that life without it would not be satisfying or even meaningful, so we try as best we can to figure out "what does it mean to be happy in my life?" or "what do I need to be happy?" We seek to describe our version of happiness—and soon realize that there is an entire spectrum of happiness experiences.

IT'S STARING US
RIGHT IN THE FACE

HERE ARE SOME things that come to mind for me when I ponder "what is happiness in my life?" I have discovered that happiness is often very simple, staring us right in the face. For me: the gift of laughter, that incredible feeling of a good laugh, releasing all the endorphins and often making my day. A feeling of contentment, sitting by a fireplace. A smile from my wife or a best friend, someone I care about, the kind that lights up the eyes. Getting absorbed by the beauty of nature, allowing time to come to a stop while I gaze at a stunning sunrise or the sparkling beauty of perfect powder snow. The feeling of blood coursing through my veins as I climb a mountain or take a hike. The sense of freedom that comes from spending time in wide-open spaces, in forests, or on mountains.

Or, alternatively, enjoying the heartbeat of a city, its vibrancy, its cafes, restaurants, and cultural events like hockey games or concerts.

The feeling of breath deep in my lungs after a good workout. Great conversation with interesting people. Being with my kids. Savouring a great meal.

A sense of celebration when my fitness club members write me about how fitness is changing their lives and knowing I have been part of that. A deep sense of satisfaction, not just in the physical sense, but in the philosophical sense, that I am doing what I most want to do in my life. (Later in the book, I'll talk more about how to do what you most want to do.)

A sense of presence, of being in the moment, of knowing that the only time I ever really have is this moment right now. One of the great lessons my life has taught me is that regret about the past and worry about the future robs us of happiness. Staying in the present allows us to uncover the happiness and contentment right under our noses, even if we're having a hard time right now. Another great lesson I have learned is that hard knocks cannot overcome happiness unless I allow them to.

HARD
KNOCKS

SO WE MAY have different ideas about what happiness is, but we know that underlying all the definitions and depictions, happiness is something that always feels good and always makes us more positive. Does that mean that an ideal happy life is one with no pain or no difficulties? No, it doesn't mean that at all. In fact, if you believe that your life cannot be happy unless you are feeling 100 percent happy 24 hours a day, then you're going to get the opposite result. You're going to make yourself feel desperately unhappy simply by trying to be happy all the time.

Life is just not like that. It isn't possible to be deliriously happy all of the time. We're all going to go through things that can make us sad or annoyed or angry or disappointed. Hard knocks are a natural part of life. The key, though, lies in what you do with the hard knocks. You have two choices: you can do nothing about them and thus stay mired in the bad feelings, or you can do something about them, either by taking some kind of action or by the way you respond emotionally. This is what experts in the field of positive psychology, one of the fastest-growing areas of modern psychology, call resilience. The ability to get back up again when something kicks the stuffing out of you. To not let the negative things define you.

My own definition of resilience is not giving up despite obstacles. If one road you're taking has a big yellow "road closed" sign on it, then go find a different road. Detours can be a lot of fun, even though you might not think so at the time. One piece of wisdom that's been around for a long time is that when something bad happens, we should figure out what the experience is teaching us. What can I learn from that mistake? In what way does a sad situation, such as the breakup of a relationship, help me understand a deeper meaning in my life? What good things might come out of the bad things?

We all want to know why some things happen. Sometimes it's good to figure this out. For example, if you're having a conflict with someone, it can be very useful to look at reasons for the conflict and what each of you is doing to contribute to it. If you want to know why you failed an exam, perhaps you need to admit that you didn't study hard enough. If you're not getting very good results from your workouts, maybe it's because you keep skipping your time at the club. If you're gaining weight, the likely reason is that you're taking in too many calories and not burning enough of them.

So, yes, there are times when we can identify a reason for negative things. Sometimes, though, things just happen at random. Sometimes it's just the luck of the draw. Sometimes the answer is in your genetics, or in your location, or just something that happens by chance. In situations like these, it isn't useful to ask why something happened. Getting stuck on "why me?" can make any unhappiness you're experiencing much worse.

Even more, that question often prevents you from doing anything about it. You don't always have to know why something happened in order for you to respond to it in a constructive and meaningful way. If I asked myself why I have arthritis, I could come up with a number of possible reasons, all of which would be sheer conjecture. Even the doctors couldn't tell me why I, Mr. Elite-Rower Fitness Guy, ended up with rheumatoid arthritis. Instead, the questions I asked myself were, "What can I do about it?" and "How can I live with this condition so it doesn't destroy my happiness and the quality of my life?"

RESILIENCE

THE FIELD OF positive psychology defines resilience, in part, as the ability to shift one's focus toward the meaningful and the positive. A resilient person focuses on solutions and problem solving, not obsessively but in a light way. It's not an exasperated "this is a crisis" followed by throwing your hands up in the air with an "Oh my God, what am I going to do?" Instead, it's "OK, this is the situation. What can I do about it?" If there's nothing you can do about it, then the question is, "How can I choose to respond to this positively?"

When people first join one of my fitness clubs, they often come with a litany of all their physical shortcomings: "I'm too fat, I'm not flexible, my knees hurt, I'm out of breath, I look ridiculous in shorts, I haven't exercised in years." I say to them, "You're telling me what isn't working in your life. Tell me instead about what is working." Even if "what works" is that the person can be on a treadmill for only five minutes before feeling winded, this means being on the treadmill for five minutes works. The person can form an intention to make it six minutes, then seven minutes.

The more we focus on what isn't working for us, then guess what? The more things are going to stop working! When you identify one thing that's not working and dwell on it, your brain will start looking for all the other things that don't work. When you get into a mood like that, all it takes is to say to yourself, "Well, what do I want to do about it—rant about it, or make it better?"

Paying attention to what is working in your life, even if they're just small things at the moment, is an absolutely key ingredient of happiness. Just recognizing a small victory in your life makes you feel happier. That's what resilience is, finding what works and then slowly increasing it—or, if something is particularly difficult and cannot be 100 percent solved, figuring out how to live with it so it doesn't damage your overall quality of life.

PRESENT
(NOT) TENSE

EARLIER I TALKED about staying in the present. When you're in the present, another quality of resilience reveals itself: a sense of flow. Have you ever become so absorbed by something that you lost all track of time? Amateur and professional athletes, writers, business people, and artists all report this feeling of being totally in the flow of the energy of what they're doing. There's something about "staying present to the present" that makes life flow better. We get through our days much more effectively if we're in the flow of the present moment than if we're caught up in regretting the past or worrying about the future.

You're not going to have a great future if you're not, right now, living in the present moment. I'm not saying that you shouldn't make plans for the future or consider the future implications of actions you might take. Because even planning happens in the present—so if you're planning something, do it with the awareness that you are still in the present. Don't let your imagination take you into living out an entire future scenario that hasn't happened yet. Besides, most of the time, future events don't conform to what we originally thought.

The other drawback of not being in the present is that it can keep you from seeing the treasures that are in front of you right now. Sometimes it's not just an escape into the future that takes us out of the present; instead we're in the present but it's a distracted present. We're not really there. I remember one time coming into a ski lodge after a great afternoon on the ski runs and sitting down at a table next to two guys who had ordered something to eat. These guys had their phones out and were texting as they sat there waiting for their food. So there they were together—friends, presumably—both communicating with other people who weren't even there. They might as well have been eating alone!

If I'm with you and I choose to text someone else and carry on an electronic conversation with that person, then I'm signaling that, at this moment, my relationship with you is not important. At the very least, I would be missing out on something very precious: the true pleasure of your company. How many great moments do we miss in life because of allowing ourselves to get distracted?

I think of my autistic daughter, Kilee. If I had not been present with her and totally focused on her during her childhood, I would not have experienced the moment when she came back into my world enough to kiss me again, hug me again . . . something that took thousands of hours to recapture. If the people who love her and care for her had not been present to her in such an unconditional way, she would have been denied a future in which she could develop to become the best she could be.

When you get home at night, are you present to your children, your spouse or partner, your roommate? Do you each talk about the day you had, or do you immediately flop down on the couch and start playing video games or texting people? Even if you live alone, you could take a few minutes just to savour being home in your quiet haven away from work with a great cup of coffee or tea, or glass of wine. There is so much happiness in those small moments around us all the time, whether we're sharing this with people or having some quiet time alone. These days we seem to have cultivated a culture of distraction rather than a culture of presence, which I think is compromising our opportunities for real happiness.

A WIDER
PERSPECTIVE

ANOTHER ASPECT OF happiness is what one philosopher recently called "living life with a wide lens." He meant looking at life with a wider perspective than just your own immediate environment. If you're sitting in your living room, look out the window and see the street or your backyard. If you're outside, look farther down the road. If you're sitting on the seashore, imagine what's beyond that horizon. One of the things I love to do when I'm skiing is to ski among trees. If I just look directly at the trees, I'm going to have a crash. Instead I need to see the whole area—the trees, the snow, the landscape—I have to take in the whole picture. I look for the opportunities, the gaps between the trees, as I ski.

Living life with a wide lens also means considering viewpoints and perspectives that are different from your own. Celebrating differences and diversities of experiences actually makes people happier than when they withdraw into their own comfortable enclaves.

Most of us are familiar with the famous Casanova—we know him as the man who wooed thousands of women. But his real claim to fame was the way in which he looked at the world. He was considered one of the most astute observers of society in his time and wrote down his observations in 12 volumes. One of the greatest pieces of advice he gave to travellers, for example, was (and I'm paraphrasing here), "When you are in a place that you have never seen before, greet it as you would greet a new friend. Let this place show you what it is, take delight in what you see, and always be ready to be surprised." Celebrating and anticipating interesting surprises: that's definitely a big part of happiness. Keep in mind, as well, the quote on the walls of many youth hostels in the world: "It doesn't matter where you go, that's where you are."

When we look at happiness from a deeper philosophical level, we are drawn to questions of meaning and purpose. The ancient Greek and Roman philosophers, such as Aristotle and Seneca, and generations of philosophers after them, as well as every religion in the world, have spent much time pondering the question "what is the good life?" They came to the conclusion that the good life is not just about pleasures and contentment. They said it is also about balance, about relationships, about the ability to think critically and clearly, about health, and about living one's life according to what they called the "virtues."

Most of us today think "virtue" means moral rectitude, even moral stuffiness, but the original meaning was about being a person of character and integrity. About pursuing the good, not just for yourself but also for others. About having the sense that life in community sometimes demands sacrifices, that we must care for the good of others. About having an orientation to life that focuses on making a difference to the world, small or large. All differences count.

On that point, it can be a big difference, such as how Martin Luther King forever changed civil rights, or how Nelson Mandela ended apartheid in South Africa. Or how Dr. Derrick MacFabe is uncovering the cause of autism (a project I am passionately involved in). Or how a young doctor founded Doctors Without Borders. Or how Johann Koss established Right To Play throughout Europe and North America. It doesn't have to be something so dramatic. It can mean working hard to raise healthy, positive children. Or treating your colleagues with respect and making them happy to work with you. Telling people that they've done good things for themselves and others creates a world of good. Large or small, virtue means making a difference through your integrity and the quality of your caring.

WHAT MATTERS
MOST

A BIG PART of happiness is to seek out the deeper parts of your own life. Think about what matters most to you and about who matters most to you. Know beyond all doubt that you can make a big difference to your family, your friends, your colleagues, your community, and even the world. Our deepest happiness will lead us to our deepest transformation, as Aristotle knew thousands of years ago and generations of philosophers and spiritual leaders have affirmed ever since.

You might ask, "Yes, but you're talking about something that not everyone can do. I mean, isn't making a difference beyond the ability of a lot of people?" Great question. Here is what modern science has found out about humans' ability to make changes toward greater happiness and fulfillment (confirming what Aristotle, in his quest for the good life, knew intuitively). Research shows that 50 percent of how we are in our lives is determined by our genetics, including our appearance, our height, our inborn temperament (some people are naturally extroverts, others are introverts, etc.). We each have a genetic heritage that determines a lot of things about us. Then 10 percent of our lives is influenced by circumstances beyond our control: where we live, our income level, our standard of living, etc.

The most important percentage is the remaining 40 percent, which is made up of circumstances that are within our control, that are susceptible to our choices and decisions. Maybe it's more like 50 percent, because living circumstances can also be changed (e.g., where you live, who you hang out with, etc.).

We have enormous potential. For example, in exercise, we know that if you increase your exercise capacity by 10 percent, you're going to get some great breakthrough results. Records are broken by increases of just tenths of seconds or less. One small action can set into motion an entire chain of improvements. If making small changes can lead to great results, think about making a 40 percent change in the circumstances you're not happy with. That's massive!

This research shows that we have a good deal more control over whether we'll be happy than we think we do. Happiness is much simpler than we think it is. We can make changes in small steps in areas that we can control as opposed to spending our time and energy worrying about what we can't control. The expression "happiness is a choice" may be overused, but it's true.

The deepest sense of happiness comes from the feeling that our life matters—matters to us and to others. Happiness is born when we realize that we don't have to be victims of circumstances, that life can offer us more freedom than we ever dreamed possible, no matter what's going on in our lives right now. That doesn't mean it all gets handed to us on a plate. Life often demands hard work and will put us through many challenges. However, we are the ones who can derive meaning from our experiences and make every experience count toward our growth. We're not wallflowers. We're out there dancing. And everyone knows that dancing makes you happy.

So let's get our bodies into the act. If we're going to be happy and healthy, we need to wake up our bodies first. We want to look good and feel good!

ONE OF OUR CLUB MEMBERS ON FITNESS AND QUALITY OF LIFE

JOHN S.

I WAS A fairly active 56-year-old self-employed maintenance worker who enjoyed an active and healthy life when, on October 13, 2011, I was involved in a motor vehicle accident that resulted in both my legs being amputated above the knee. I spent four months in various hospitals recovering and regaining some health back and being taught how to prepare myself for my new life challenges.

It was suggested that I join a gym to help me build my upper body strength, as I would need it for transfers when not wearing my prosthetics, and to gain overall body strength because having the prostheses on puts added stress on my body.

It was an excellent suggestion and that's exactly what happened. I decided on a personal trainer and it was a great call—totally the right thing to do! I have an exercise routine that has helped me in my new circumstances. My trainer is quite knowledgeable in a variety of aspects involving the body, how it moves, and how it should be trained at different times. And all the nutrition talks help, too!

Overall, I have increased endurance, balance, and

coordination, and have added a fair amount of muscle to my upper half. Also, the rotator issue that I had before my accident has been fixed by working with my trainer. The fitness professionals who have worked with me have always been cordial and are regularly there to say hello and comment on my constant progress, especially when I first started to walk in my prosthetics.

I've mentioned many times to family and friends that GoodLife has been very good for my quality of life, and I look forward to what comes next.

CHAPTER THREE

LOOKING
GOOD

WHEN IT COMES to fitness, the human body is a pleasure-seeking organism. We'll do it only if it feels good. However, the desire to feel good isn't what initially motivates most people to try exercise. Most people join a fitness club because they don't like the way they look and want to look better. Given how our culture values physical appearance, it's small wonder that very few of us are completely happy with the bodies we have. There's nothing wrong with wanting to look good. In this chapter I want to see if we can tap into this very human desire to be attractive and appealing to others as a way of getting to the more important and lasting reasons to pursue regular fitness activities.

Looking good requires a healthy balance between your body type and your self-image, whereas a good weight needs to be customized to what is appropriate for you and what improves your functionality. These two aspects may not be in sync. Popular media throughout history have often promoted "perfect" stereotypes, trying to influence men and women to achieve these ideal bodies. So a woman may look in the mirror and think, "I'm fat," when in fact her body weight may be exactly what it's supposed to be.

On the other end of the scale, a man might look in the mirror and see not a hulk with muscles coming out of his earlobes, but a skinny guy who is scared to walk down the beach, and he might decide to take drugs to bulk up. Just as a woman may feel that being thin will make people think more highly of her, a man feels that bigger muscles will make people think more highly of him.

All of this happens because we've bought into cultural ideals of "female beauty" and "manliness" that are not based in the reality of who we are.

BECOME THE
10 YOU ARE

THERE WAS A movie back in 1979 called "*10*"—a romantic comedy starring actress Bo Derek as the epitome of physical perfection. It was trendsetting at the time, and the expression "being a 10" entered popular speech. Suddenly everyone was trying to decide who was a 10 and who wasn't. Initially it meant that if you ranked among this exclusive set, you were physically perfect: spectacularly good-looking, spectacularly fit. So what does being a 10 mean?

Well, at that time the female was the focus, thanks to the "sex goddess" mentality. Today's films and television series have created an equal expectation that both male and female roles will be played by actors with perfect bodies. Think of the "shirtless" phenomenon that's so familiar in the entertainment world now, whether it's James Bond striding out of the water displaying his abs or male vampires sporting their perfect torsos.

Well, I want to stand the "10" idea on its head by suggesting that being a 10 is a process of *becoming*, of moving toward creating a truly good life on all fronts. It's *not* about perfection, and it isn't even about accomplishing goals or competing to be a star at something. It's about giving up perfection as a goal and instead taking a journey through your life that is a "10" journey, a pathway of committing to be the best you can be—*you,* the individual *you,* not the image projections of popular magazines or TV. If, every day, you can say to yourself, "I am moving toward better health, more happiness, and boundless energy," and really believe that and act on it, then you're a 10.

If I were to meet you tomorrow, what would I see about you? How do you want people to see you? Most importantly, how do you see yourself? That goes a long way toward determining what other people will see in you. In other words, you get to influence people's perception of you by making a decision about how you want to see yourself. If you see yourself in a positive light—if you celebrate all the daily victories that contribute to the good life—then people are going to relate to your positive vibe. They will experience you as a person radiating better health, more happiness, and boundless energy. They will see a 10.

I have to say that I've never met a person who exercises regularly who is not a 10. Fit people tend to have lots of energy. They walk with a bounce in their step. They have shining eyes and great posture. They hold their bodies in an upright yet fluid position, and there's confidence in their stride. Their skin has a healthy glow, and you can just feel their resilience and their optimism toward life. At the end of a long, busy day, the fit person is the one who still has a spark of energy. If I see a person take the stairs quickly and lightly, I know they exercise regularly, whether by working out or embracing an active lifestyle.

A few years back, we surveyed our GoodLife members to find out how they felt about their lifestyle and overall sense of well-being. At the time we were supporting an Adopt-A-Doc initiative to address a shortage of doctors, so we also wanted to find out if our members had adequate access to a physician. Over 3,000 of our members responded, most indicating that, on average, they worked out three times a week. For fun, since the survey was done around Valentine's Day, we asked them to rank what qualities, either physical or personality traits, made a person most attractive to them. The top responses were not broad shoulders or shapely legs or hair colour or even body type. Overwhelmingly they zeroed in on a positive attitude, a confident bearing, a great smile, a sense of humour. The respondents also strongly expressed that people who appear to take care of themselves are attractive.

Almost three-quarters of the respondents—72 percent—said that feeling at home in their body boosts their self-esteem. Two-thirds—66 percent—said they felt it was important to maintain the sense of their own attractiveness as they age. The commitment to maintaining their own confidence levels and well-being—the hallmarks of a great attitude—was a major factor in why they continued with fitness, why they made physical activity an important part of their life.

People who are comfortable in their own bodies and with themselves as whole persons—body, mind, and soul—make others feel at ease, and, as a result, they draw people to them. Other people like to be in their presence. One of the highest compliments I think we can give to others is "I feel good when I'm around you." That's a 10 in my mind.

You know, I think we have a society right now that still wants to make people focus on their flaws. To me that's a complete waste of time. It's also a fact that what we think are our flaws often aren't flaws at all! How often have you focused on one of your so-called flaws only to have someone compliment you on that very thing? Let's say you have really curly hair that's difficult to "tame" and you see that as a flaw. Then you meet someone who says, "I just love your curly hair!"

Take a moment now to think about what you get complimented for. When I present a seminar or workshop at conferences around the world, I often ask people—all strangers to each other—to get into small groups and talk about what they admire about one another, right off the bat. This exercise in awareness of how others see us can be a real eye-opener. People often gain insight into themselves that they never thought of before. For example, someone might say, "I didn't think I had a great laugh, but she seems to really like the way I laugh." Or, "I never really considered that wearing red looks good on me until a complete stranger said to me, 'That colour looks great on you . . . you seem so alive and energized.'"

Typically I then get everyone to chant "I'm a 10" vigorously, repeatedly, standing on chairs until their voices fill with confidence, and everyone is laughing together. I've even seen this work with bankers and accountants, believe it or not!

As I've mentioned, being a 10 is a journey, not a destination. That's why my idea of "10-ness" fits so well with something else I always say: "Good enough is good enough." As I said above, it's about moving every day toward better health, more happiness, and boundless energy. If you're doing that, then every day good enough is good enough, right here and now in the present. Toss out the perception that 10 means perfect and replace it with the idea that 10 means feeling vibrantly alive in the moment, in the next moment, and in the moment after that.

I know I tend to talk a lot about giving up the idea of perfection. First of all, perfection is never possible. So why do we use perfection to beat ourselves up with, or to diminish who we truly are? I have never met a person who thinks he or she has a perfect body. And that's a good thing! Getting into shape is never about attaining perfection—perfection is a complete illusion. Being a 10 is about becoming the very best you can be. Best *never* means perfect. Feeling vibrantly alive *is* being a 10. Exercise can give you an inner and outer radiance that makes people notice you. You'll look good by looking like *you* at your very best in the present moment, by feeling comfortable inside your skin, and by heightening your aliveness as a human being!

You are a 10 and that's good enough!

YOUR BODY TYPE
DETERMINES
HOW YOU LOOK

LOOKING GOOD IS about being comfortable in your own skin and realizing that your body type, what scientists call your somatotype, determines much of the way you look. Even if you totally accept your body type and make your body the best for that type, you will never reach "perfection." Good news: you can get 95 percent of what you want with half an hour of exercise three times a week.

There are three main body types: ectomorph, endomorph, and mesomorph. Ectomorphs are linear. They tend to be tall, with long limbs and a slender trunk; they have a smaller chest frame, hip girdle, and hipbones; and they have narrow shoulders. Endomorphs are rounder overall, or they have round thighs, round arms, a round face, and a round chest. Mesomorphs have a larger chest, smaller hips, and large shoulders, and seem to be muscular without doing anything. People are actually a combination of these different types, but most tend to be predominantly one type.

When it comes to exercising, ectomorphs gain some muscle and become stronger, endomorphs lose some roundness and put on some muscle, and mesomorphs become more dramatically muscular.

Furthermore, these different body types excel at different sports. Endomorphs or mesomorphs may be better at swimming because they have more body fat to help support them in the water, but long, linear ectomorphs will flourish as rowers—that's me!

EVOLUTION
PLAYS A ROLE

YOU CAN'T FIGHT Mother Nature. Genetically, males and females have differing tendencies. Historically, at least until the Industrial Revolution, females tended to be the gatherers of food. They didn't run as much, and they bore children. They carried the loads of food and children, so heavier hips became a physical adaptation over thousands of years.

As a result of this evolutionary pattern, women came to carry fat first and foremost on their derrières and their thighs, where it didn't interfere with gathering food or having children. When a woman didn't have reliable food sources, those were the safest parts of her body to store fat.

Which is why these are the first places where a woman tends to put on weight and why these seem to be the most stubborn places to lose weight. If you're a woman, and you've got extra weight on your abdomen, it can be lost quite easily, but you'll go crazy waiting for it to come off your derrière.

Now let's look at men. The average man carries extra weight on his abdomen. Thousands of years ago men were hunters. They had to be able to run, either toward something or away from something. The best place to store fat and not have it interfere with running is the stomach. And if an attacker couldn't be outrun, men had all that fat protecting the vital organs that are also in that area of the body. The second place a man puts on weight is his back, where it also acts as protection and doesn't get in the way. Given that men did so much with their upper body, such as hitting, punching, or throwing, nature made sure they didn't store fat on their arms.

By the way, so many men want to have a "washboard stomach," showing all their abdominal muscles, but for the average male, getting to that point means he has about 6 to 8 percent body fat. Some men would have to go to 4 percent, which is too low. A small number of men can show those muscles at 10 percent body fat. What men need to realize is that they won't get those "perfect abs" until their body fat, as a whole, is low and they've toned up their whole bodies. This is nearly impossible for many men, and some endanger their health by reducing their body fat to too low a level.

The key thing for all of us is to shift our motivation from looking good to please others to looking good to please ourselves. We've got it backwards in this society. We seek to impress others, but we're not impressed with ourselves. If you can make yourself happy and comfortable in your own body, in most cases what other people think won't matter.

One of the things about "looking good" that can really bug us is the anxiety we have about other people judging our appearance (or our exercise routine). People often tell me they don't want to join a fitness club because they're afraid of being looked at. "I don't want to look foolish next to all those buff guys," they say, or "I don't look good in shorts," or "look at her—her movement has flow, and she never misses a beat, but I'm always lagging behind."

I learned firsthand that the most useless question you can ask yourself is "who's looking?" One day when I was working out in one of my clubs, I thought that, since I was the owner, I would immediately be recognized by the members. That made me self-conscious, because I don't have perfect technical form when I exercise. "Oh, they're going to expect me to do this perfectly because I'm supposed to be Mr. Fitness Guy," I thought. To my surprise, when I looked around to see what others were looking at, I saw that no one was looking at me! Everyone was far too busy with their own exercise programs. They were looking at the displays on their treadmills, at the instructor in front of a class, or at their personal trainer. This gave me the freedom to just relax and go ahead with my own routine.

When you just work with the body type you are, accept your somatotype, and just go with it, you can stop worrying about other people looking at you and have the freedom to enjoy your life.

TWO COMPONENTS
OF LOOKING GOOD

THERE ARE TWO components of looking good.

The first is feeling good about yourself just for participating in physical activity, feeling good about every improvement you make, as opposed to thinking you'll look good only when you're perfect. When I was training for the 1980 Olympics, I was in the best shape of my life. I weighed 215 pounds with 8 percent body fat. However, I worked out six hours a day, I ate like crazy, slept a lot, and that's all I did. There was no way I could do any of the other things I wanted to do. For most of us, that trade-off in the pursuit of a perfect body is just not workable. The key to looking good is being prepared to thank yourself for every improvement you make, to see yourself in the mirror and know you look as good as you did last year—which means you're actually slowing down the effects of aging.

The second component of looking good is what goes into people saying to you, "You look good"—the strength to have good posture, the cardiovascular capacity to not look tired, and the flexibility in your joints so you don't become old before your time. The act of exercising creates energy, and as you create energy, you give your body vitality. And if you have vitality, you look good.

This is the great paradox: if you stop worrying about people looking at you and just go ahead with your exercise, realizing that no one is going to judge you for your form (other than your personal trainer!), that's when you'll get that glow, that posture, that energy . . . and people will say to you, "Hey, you look good." Exercise can take you all the way from wondering "who's looking?" to hoping they are.

What happens when you get fit is that you become comfortable with yourself. As that comfort level goes up, you gradually transform yourself into what you want to be, within your own capabilities. You're exercising and all of a sudden your muscles feel firmer, you hold your head a little higher, your posture improves, your joints are aligned, and you carry your weight better—even if it's the same weight you had when you began. Your skin starts to get better. Your respiration improves. Exercise speeds up the elimination of toxins from your body.

When you exercise, you take oxygen into your lungs, your blood picks up the oxygen, and your heart pumps that clean blood through your arteries (the arteries oxygenate your blood). The veins take the blood minus the oxygen back to the lungs to be renewed. Through exercise, your arteries and veins expand and contract with greater elasticity. Exercise burns up some of the waste products created by various bodily functions. As it burns them up, it cleans your arteries and veins, and the blood moves more easily. And your lungs take in oxygen more efficiently. You get more fresh air to your head and body. As a result, you can think better. (We'll talk later about the correlation between exercise and intelligence.) Your body functions as the active human being you are.

EVERY PART IS
MEANT FOR EXERCISE

EVERY PART OF your body is meant for exercise. Your body is meant to function, not just to be passive. Say, for example, you're not that physically active, and one night you go out to a party and dance the night away. When you're back home and having a nice warm shower, chemicals called endorphins kick into your bloodstream—your body's way of saying, "I'm making you feel good because I'm hoping you'll do this again tomorrow." While you were dancing, you burned off some of the negative, stress-producing chemicals in your body.

After you break the cycle of inactivity, sometime between six weeks and six months later you will start to feel the pleasure of exercise, and your body will tell you, "This is good." Why, then, doesn't that night of dancing make you run right out and join a fitness club or buy some exercise equipment for your home? The reason lies again in our evolutionary patterns. For most of our history, we often didn't have enough food, or at least a consistent supply of food. We evolved to store and conserve fat so we would have it when we needed it. On top of that, generations ago, all of life was physically demanding.

This not an issue anymore—most of us don't have to worry about starvation, and we don't get enough activity. In fact, in North America we usually have to worry about the opposite—overeating. The point is that our bodies are still in the "conserve energy" mode. When we're sitting on the couch being sedentary, we slip back into the mode of "there might be a hurricane tomorrow, and maybe I won't be able to get food, so I'd better save my energy." Yet your body is filled with the survival chemicals needed for fight or flight from eons ago.

We need to evolve a bit further! The fact of the matter is that since we do have enough food, the very act of doing something physical creates more energy. That activity burns off those fight-or-flight chemicals the way nature designed us to do.

That's why exercise makes us feel energetic. It's self-perpetuating. We all think the remedy for stress is to relax. But physical activity creates the energy so we can relax. It's a paradox: Be active and you will relax more deeply. Stay on the couch and your relaxation will simply make you more tired.

The big challenge in looking good for your body type is beating your habitual urge to do nothing. Become a participant in life instead of a victim avoiding starvation. The key issue in looking good is realizing you will never be totally satisfied with how you look. Don't get caught on the perfection treadmill. You'll drive yourself crazy, and you'll quit. Then you'll never break the bad habit of inactivity.

At age 45, it is possible, through regular physical activity, to get back the physique you had when you were 25. At 45, as opposed to 25, you take longer to recover from exercise, and you have to be more consistent about doing it. Whereas a 25-year-old can miss a week of exercise and not notice a difference, a 45-year-old will have to maintain a routine every other day. Long-term conditioning will accomplish a lot. In terms of looking good, regular exercise is going to help you look good a lot longer.

As you get older, you lose, on average, half a pound of muscle a year. If you stay fit, you won't lose it, or you'll lose a lot less. By staying fit and strong, you also reduce your resting heart rate, which will give you a greater cardiovascular capacity than most people your age.

In this culture it's not realistic to think that you're not going to get caught in the "looking good" mindset. Recognize that everyone thinks about it, and you're not alone in that. This doesn't mean you have to kill yourself over it. Realize that, as much as everyone wants to look perfect, the real goal is to be the best you can be for your life and to insist that you get that by exercising three times a week for 30 minutes.

DON'T MAKE THE PROCESS TOO HARD

WHEN I FIRST started in the fitness business in 1979, my background was as an athlete, and I had also experienced intense rehabilitation after my motorcycle accident. I thought the only way to exercise was "no pain, no gain." When people came to join my first club, I'd take them through the equipment and push them so hard that some of them took days to recover from their sore muscles.

One day I hired a new accountant, Bill Shanks (who is still my accountant). At the time Bill was a very fit 29-year-old—a basketball player. I insisted that my accountant join my club. As was my practice, whenever someone new joined, I followed up with a call two or three days later to see how it was going. I had noticed that Bill didn't come in for his second workout, so I phoned him to find out why.

"I can't get out of bed," he said. "I'm too sore."

"This isn't good," I thought, and I changed the whole strategy. I realized that when you push someone so hard that he or she collapses under the strain, you're "training to failure." From that point on, I decided to train people only to success.

When we put people on the equipment now, we first look at their joint function. We want to make sure they experience the equipment with their whole range of motion. A full range of motion is important because the number one reason people get old is that they lose flexibility. We start them off with exercise they can manage for the whole range of motion. Invariably most people can lift more weight in a short range of motion, but only half the weight with a full range of motion. For example, they can easily lift a 20-pound box of groceries from their hips to their chest, but struggle with the full range of motion of picking it up off the floor and putting it over their head.

Another reason we want people to go through the whole range of motion is that they are less likely to get injured when they're strong throughout their whole range of motion. We know, for example, that 80 percent of back injuries are caused by weak muscles.

Once people start doing exercises through their full range of motion, they can increase the weights really quickly.

What does this have to do with looking good? If you're exercising using your whole range of motion, within your first month you will start to build muscle. As research shows, the metabolic rate of muscles is much faster than the metabolic rate of organs. If you exercise regularly, you're going to get some good results muscle-wise. As you gain muscle, you'll look better and burn fat because those new muscles are burning off more calories.

Often people who come in to exercise say, "My weight hasn't changed." What they've actually done is lose two pounds of fat and put on two pounds of muscle. People who have more muscle burn more calories even at rest. Less activity means you slow down your body's ability to burn calories. More activity, as I said, burns more calories. Muscle takes up less space than fat and looks better. That's why fit people tend to look better longer. You will have more energy. All around, muscle makes your life easier.

Looking good in terms of having more muscle gives you benefits far beyond your appearance. There is less physical stress on the body. If you are capable of moving 100 pounds on a back machine and then you have to pick up 30 pounds of groceries, that's only 30 percent of what you are capable of. Your chances of getting injured are lower. The same thing happens with flexibility. If you're flexible enough to stretch to get a coffee cup from the top shelf of your cupboard, your life is less stressful. Or if your child grabs and pulls you, you won't pull a muscle. Injuries happen when you're weaker.

Statistics show that fit people live a minimum of two years longer than the average population. I believe it is much longer. But what statisticians don't talk about is quality of life. If you can dance 10 dances in a row and not be winded, isn't that pleasurable? If you never need to worry about what's in the grocery bag because you can lift it and not hurt yourself, doesn't that make your life easier? If you can live doing what you want to do instead of worrying about it, isn't that much more fun? All these things equip you to handle life. It makes a difference for the people you love, as well as in your work and in your play, to be fit.

THE GLOW OF
HEALTH AND
WELL-BEING

IF YOU GIVE your body a total fitness program—one that is easy to do—you're not going to put on more weight, and you're going to have a lot more energy. Looking good becomes feeling good, and it leads to longevity and quality of life. If I could get only one message across in this chapter, it would be this: There are no rights or wrongs about looking good; there is only what's right for you and your body type. Don't look at someone else and decide she's "right" and you're "wrong." You'll find that, as you get fit, you become more at home in your body. You'll start to look good because you're radiating confidence from within. You'll have the glow of good health and well-being, and people will find that attractive.

I like to say that exercise is a form of self-respect. If you look after your own health, it means you're capable of being involved with others. Jimmy Buffett has a song about people who have "nothing to share, like driving around with no spare." If you're taxed physically and emotionally, you're driving around without a spare. You may have a "spare tire" of fat, but you won't have that extra energy and vitality for yourself and others.

The body is absolutely phenomenal. It can do wonders. Most people can achieve a fitness level they would never dream possible. Ninety-nine percent of people can do things they don't believe they can do. I didn't really get into skiing until I was 39 years old, and I had rheumatoid arthritis. I've been heli-skiing now (the helicopter drops you in fresh powder at the top of a mountain) for more than 20 years, despite my arthritis. You can do so much. A person who hasn't walked a block can be walking five miles six months later.

The body wants exercise so badly. It needs it, craves it, and it rewards you when you do it, by making you look good and feel good. There isn't anything you can spend your money on that does as much for you as exercise. There isn't a medication you can buy, or a car, or a house, or a trip that will make you feel the way you do when your body is fit and healthy.

As I said at the beginning of this chapter, most people start to exercise because of the way they look, but after six months or so, they stay with it because of the way they feel. Self-acceptance, self-awareness, and fitness are a happiness circle. When that circle is complete, and you're moving around it every day with a light, fit step, people will come up to you and say, "Wow! You look really good!"

SOME OF OUR
CLUB MEMBERS
ON LOOKING GOOD

JULIE M.

ALL OF MY life I have struggled with being overweight and have been incredibly self-conscious about my appearance. As a child, I wasn't very physically active. I didn't want to participate in any sports because I didn't think I would be good enough because of my weight. I also developed poor eating habits and became an emotional eater—relying on food for comfort or as a reward.

In my mid-teens, I lost some weight by changing my eating habits and exercising. However, I gradually reverted to my old ways and allowed the weight to pile on again. I finally reached a point where I weighed 247 pounds and had almost accepted that I would be obese the rest of my life.

Knowing diabetes, heart disease, and cancer ran in my family made it scary for me to think about my future. I was always exhausted and had frequent headaches and back pain. I didn't believe I could do anything to change my health. In August 2012, I joined a GoodLife club and began to see a new, positive path for my life that I could choose to take. I was nervous about going to a new gym, but all of the staff were so welcoming and encouraging. Right from the start, I began to see changes, and I began to believe in myself too, and to take control of my life! I have been given the skills I need to safely and effectively work out, and I have developed a more positive relationship with food.

In July 2014, a few days before my wedding, I reached my goal and now have lost 103 pounds, 73.75 inches, and 24 percent body fat. I have gone from wearing a size 20 to a size 6. With every new challenge, I gain more confidence. I am capable of so much!

On my wedding day, I walked down the aisle in a gown that I never dreamed I would be able to wear, toward a future with many new and exciting possibilities.

RICH B.

IT'S NOT MY being overweight or underweight that stopped my progression toward health. It was the distance between laziness and willpower. If only the future could be changed with minimal effort, my laziness could rule time. My minimal effort had cruelly proven to be a poor theory, as I could not see my toes in the shower anymore. I would look at my stomach and be awestruck by its sheer magnificence—it was huge. I was not impressed. If I decided to trash my stomach, I was going to have to lift a finger—not my idea of overwhelming excitement, although I was not about to buy a backup beeper for my big butt.

So—my brain decided to join GoodLife. My body decided not to join GoodLife. The two of them argued and argued over and over for I don't know how long. The two of them were really ticking me off.

I looked at the treadmill and thought, "I could do that," while my body was yelling, "Don't get me on that devil-made torture machine!" But I did, because I rarely listen to my body, and why should I? It doesn't know what it's doing anyway.

Then I looked at the weights and thought, "I could do that, too." In time-stopping horror, my body was screaming, "Have you lost it? Are you insane? Don't you touch those things!" Once again, my brain won the war and I continued to disregard my body's request for freedom. The easy thing to do would be to quit, go home, lie on the couch, eat ice cream, and watch TV.

It's several years later, and I've continued to work out. I can see significant shrinkage—in my stomach, that is. The moral of the story: I don't know. You'll have to figure that out on your own. All I know is that I have more energy now, I'm stronger, and I feel better about myself. Now go away and do something!

AVRIL F.

BIG. THAT WAS me—bigger than I wanted to be for as long as I can remember. Not fat, not exactly. I could always carry a little more weight than some people because, on me, the weight did not all collect at my waist or my butt. It spread out everywhere. I had big arms, a big neck, and big thighs—I was just too big.

My diet seemed fine and when I tried fad diets I might lose a little weight. But soon it would be back. I seemed active enough. Heck, back in high school I even made the school basketball team.

Being big never really held me back. I just wished I could be smaller. I had a good marriage and a great family. I graduated from law school and built a busy law practice. I was the model superwoman with the world by the tail and an extra 25 pounds.

One day I was referred to a surgeon. She dealt with my health problem and then said I needed to start a comprehensive and disciplined program of regular exercise. I started to explain how that wouldn't be necessary, how active I was, how I wasn't really fat—I'd been big as long as I could remember. When I stopped talking, she explained how that wasn't the same as an overall workout that was available at the fitness centre she attended. She even offered to take me to her club and she introduced me to everyone there.

At first it was awful. I could only work out for a few minutes at a time and only at the lowest settings on the equipment. Tiny 18-year-old girls, a little bigger than my daughter, and 60-year-old women, who could almost be my mother, could outshine me. It both embarrassed and inspired me. I never really knew I was in such bad shape.

Soon I could last a little longer and at higher levels. After a few weeks I went with my family for our regular bike ride. Instead of my husband and kids riding off into the distance and then stopping to wait for me, this time they stayed with me. Then it suddenly struck me that I was keeping up with them!

With my law practice I couldn't work out in the evenings consistently, so I learned to get up an hour earlier and exercise to start my day. Soon I wasn't tired anymore because I was sleeping better. I started to feel good for the first time in my life. I got into a pretty consistent pattern of 20 to 25 workouts every month. I felt better and better. I often worked out with my doctor friend and she taught me things about nutrition and lifestyle. Even my husband and children became healthier.

As the weeks and months progressed, so did I. That first fall I was having a terrible time in my favourite stores finding clothes that fit properly, and I realized that I couldn't wear plus sizes any more. My husband cheerfully helped me mark and pin my old clothes, and armloads of garments had to be taken in. He began to tell me that I looked great. I kept a pair of my old pants and tried them on every once in a while, just to marvel at the changes.

Working out became so enjoyable that I began to dread going on vacation because I would miss my exercise. I got really good at finding other clubs to use when I was out of town.

I had always thought it was normal to feel bad all the time, exhausted all the time. I always expected to die at a relatively young age, like many of my relatives. Not anymore. The other night, as I was trying on some of my new, slim clothes in front of my new, full-length mirrors, my husband and I were talking about things we would do well into our retirement. I'm only in my 40s, but the way I feel now, I expect to live forever.

When I look in the mirror now, I marvel at how my life has changed. Reflected back is not a big person. It's not me plus 25 pounds. It's not me dressing to look thinner. The reflection is just me. The small me I always wanted to be.

Just me. I like that.

CHAPTER FOUR

FEELING GOOD

THE REASON PEOPLE keep exercising—the reason they like to be fit—is really only partly about how they look. This is perhaps only 25 percent of the equation, even though looking good, as we've been talking about it, is often the primary motivator to get them exercising in the first place. Seventy-five percent of the equation is how they feel. The best way to describe it is to refer to the lack of feeling good. An athlete, or someone else who has always been active, will say, "Do you remember how it felt so good when we scored that touchdown/won that race/painted the whole house in one day?" and so forth. A person who has never been fit doesn't have that memory of "how it felt so good."

So I ask people who have never been active, "Have you ever been sick?" Most people have had the flu. If I asked what it was like they would probably answer, "I felt terrible. I had low energy. I had such aches and pains." Well, that's what it's like being unfit. However, unlike the flu, it doesn't just hit you out of the blue. "Unfitness" happens slowly, insidiously, so you don't really notice.

Let's take alcohol consumption as an example. If someone

gets drunk, the hangover feels terrible. You do it for a week, and it feels really terrible. You do it for a year, and it's "the way life is." You habituate to feeling bad, and you think that's normal. Your functional level is like a hangover. It's an "unfit-over." Your body knows it should have energy and vitality, but your brain and body learn to accept a lower quality of life.

Or try this: imagine that you have had allergies all your life, and your nose is always stuffed up. Then imagine that one day, all of a sudden, you wake up and you don't have the sniffles anymore. You can breathe. You can smell that apple pie baking. You can smell the lilac bushes. That's what being fit is like. For a fit person, the sun is shining. You go to the store and you have extra energy. You spring up the stairs. You talk to someone, and you have extra enthusiasm. That's feeling good. It didn't happen because you sat and read a couple of books on self-esteem. It happened because your body is functioning as it should be, and this puts you—body, mind, and soul—into a state of well-being.

If, in contrast, your fitness level declines into unfitness, you keep noticing things you can't do. You become wrapped up in not wanting to do something that would expose your weakness. You don't go swimming because you don't want people to see your belly. You don't play squash because you get winded. The fun you would get from waterskiing, or hiking, or playing with your grandchildren, or running with your dog—all that is part of feeling good. You can't do any of these things if your low energy levels have you slouching on the couch.

When you exercise for 30 minutes three times a week, life suddenly becomes so much "tastier." There is a chemical reaction in your body that tells you physical activity is the right thing to do. You don't need to know the biochemistry of endorphins to know that they make you feel good and that they are triggered by exercise. Exercising is unbelievably easy. All you need to do, three times a week, is raise your heart rate enough so when you're talking, you're gasping a little bit for breath—not choking for breath, just gasping. All you need to do, three times a week, is make your muscles a little stronger than they were by means of what we call a progressive overload system. You'll notice within six weeks how much better you feel.

ISN'T EXERCISE BORING?

MOST PEOPLE FEEL better right away for one huge reason: self-control. They have taken control of their bodies. If you just relax and listen to your body, it will tell you what it needs in order to feel good. However, you may ask, what about the fact that—after six weeks or six months—exercise may become routine, or you might lose motivation?

When people say they get tired of exercise, there are two reasons. One is that they have gone beyond "good enough is good enough" and just push and push until they can't push any more. Anyone would get tired of always pushing. So say, "Good enough is good enough."

The other reason is a feeling of boredom. People ask, "How can I run the same route three times a week? How can I run on a treadmill? How can I lift the same weights?" Two answers to that. First, I say we are very lucky because there are so many ways to change up our exercise routines, both indoors and outdoors. Nature itself is always changing, so that alone can add new interest. Second, for all the benefits we get from exercise, just plain decide to enjoy it. Accept the routine, like brushing your teeth, eating, sleeping. It's a necessity of life.

If you exercise outside, nature makes it such a wonderful place—running on the beach when the sand is piled up from a storm, walking through falling leaves, or shoveling snow. I love to watch people on the street or in the parks skateboarding, biking, shooting hoops, or power walking. Wherever you are, you can find delight in your surroundings. See that half hour three times a week as a time to become mindful of and alive to your surroundings. If you're lucky enough to go to a club that has a variety of facilities, you can use the display screens on the exercise equipment for feedback. It is motivating to watch your heart rate zone as you work out, to see how many calories you are burning, or how far you have cycled, or how efficient your strokes are on a rowing machine. You can plug in your iPod and listen to your favourite music. You can tune in to television monitors, some integrated right into your piece of equipment.

Sometimes there is a place for doing nothing. Just let your brain float and be aware of whatever thoughts float into your mind and out again. That's what happens in meditation. In meditation you clear the mind and let it float. Exercise can be a form of moving meditation. In giving yourself a little "me" time, you can turn your attention inward while you're exercising and lower your stress level. Many people these days practice BodyFlow or other forms of yoga. You can bring this same mind state to many forms of exercising.

DISTINGUISH BETWEEN EXERCISE AND SPORT

I HAVE HEARD from many people over the years that one reason they don't feel good about exercising is a lack of confidence. They have in their mind a "failure syndrome" created by some experience years ago of not being successful at school in a team sport when they felt they didn't measure up. They associate exercise as leading to some sport and, often, competition. Sport is descended from fun and play, with rules that further help enjoyment. It becomes sport when winning is the goal. Instead of trying to win, just focus on showing up, just to "do." Just to move. Maybe be playful with it. Yes, you need a certain intensity for results. After a while, you can just enjoy it, having happier, easier, and medium workouts. Be nice to yourself. Pat yourself on the back, often. Showing up is the most important part of fitness: no opponents, and everything is a win.

I am very encouraged by the change in this landscape. Today many school boards are placing a big focus on physical literacy. That was not in evidence when I founded our GoodLife Kids Foundation in 1998. Many teachers and schools are now introducing functional fitness to improve physical literacy—with an overarching goal of fostering healthy, active living. Schools are getting students active in creative and fun ways, such as through fitness circuits that use exercise tubing, or bi-weekly off-site visits to local fitness facilities.

As adults, it is important we shed any feelings of judgment—any residual feelings of "I don't measure up." Instead, revel in the fact that you are exercising and taking care of your health.

FITNESS DOESN'T
REQUIRE SKILL

When you get to the point where you do decide to go to a fitness club or buy a piece of exercise equipment, or you resolve to take a brisk walk every evening, give yourself a big round of applause just for showing up in your own life and taking control. Next, realize that the activities you need for fitness are non-athletic. They do not require skill. Not one activity you need to do for fitness requires special skill. If you can hold a pen, if you can brush your teeth, if you can open a book, you can do fitness activities.

The simplest form of exercise is walking. Almost everyone can walk (unless you have a disability that makes walking impossible). If you go for a walk on a regular basis for half an hour, five times a week, that alone will make you a lot fitter than most of your friends and colleagues. It will strengthen your arteries, lower your fatty acids, regulate your blood pressure, and help you control your weight.

If you want to help your heart, as well, you need to go further and be active in a way that gets your heart rate up into what we call the training zone, three times a week, for 12 to 20 minutes. You can do that by walking really fast. You can do it by jogging. You can ride a stationary bicycle at home or at a club. This requires no learning curve. If you have two legs that can move, we can put you on a bicycle and you will know how to do it. You can do the same thing by walking on a treadmill or using a piece of equipment called a cross-trainer. You can learn how to use a cross-trainer in under five minutes. Some equipment may have a longer learning curve, perhaps half an hour, but none of it is rocket science in terms of learning how to use it.

For strength training, you can be taught how to do a push-up in two minutes and a sit-up in one minute. If you go to a club, most of them have strength-training equipment where all you have to do is move pins to change the weight. You can learn to use the strength-training machines in less than half an hour.

Fitness facilities have nothing to do with being athletic. You will see many athletes at fitness clubs, some of them elite, training for specific sports. For the average person, though, fitness is mostly about making their body function the way it was intended to, so their brain will function the way it was meant to, so they get the most and the best out of life.

IT'S SO
EASY

THE PROBLEM IS that we take our bodies for granted. We just assume we will be healthy and don't have to do anything to guarantee that we stay healthy. When we get sick or have an accident, we realize we can't take our bodies for granted. Sometimes it is sickness or adversity that brings us to the pursuit of fitness (more on that later in this book).

The reality is that, in terms of our fitness and health, we're born with the opportunity to be everything we can be. Over thousands of years of evolution, nature has made it easy to do what it takes in order to feel good. You have 168 hours in a week. Your body will function fantastically if you devote an hour and a half to two hours of that 168 to your fitness. Two hours a week is 104 hours a year—4.3 days—spent on exercise. Assuming the average person lives 78 years, 335 days of your life would be devoted to exercise. It's been proven that you gain two years or more if you exercise regularly. Let's assume that you get 10 or 15 more years of quality-of-life longevity from doing fitness activities on a regular basis throughout your adult life. Think of the payoff. At the least, it's more than 100 percent. Can you think of any other investment that will give you that?

People often ask me, "If all this is true, then why in our

culture are most people so abysmally unfit?" We have to consider that the "unfitness epidemic," with its chronic anxiety, fatigue, and feelings of unease, is really only a blip on the human radar screen of history. It's only been about 50 years since people didn't have to do something physical every day. The ease of life we have today in the Western world is relatively recent. Our evolutionary concept of needing physical activity hasn't caught up. Twenty percent of the population is aware and does physical activity. The other 80 percent knows, but is not doing it. About 17 percent of the total population of the United States and Canada is working out at fitness clubs. Many are doing other things; probably 30 percent get enough activity from a healthy lifestyle. This percentage is gradually rising by 1 to 2 percent a year.

We used to get so much exercise in times past that it wore us out. We would die young from years of 16-hour days in the coalmines or in the fields. That's not the case today. Now we have to exercise so as not to rust out from inactivity. Work has changed to become less physically challenging but more mentally stressful. I think a time is coming when more people will become smart enough to realize this is what they have to do, especially when they discover it doesn't have to be hard—that it's actually very easy. It's actually fun.

Think about eating. You know you need to eat. The gnawing in your stomach when you're hungry tells you that. And if you don't eat for a few weeks, you die. What happens when you don't exercise is that you're hastening your death— your death is "making haste slowly." While you're hastening your death, you're lowering your quality of life because you'll be more tired and feel less vital.

To get people to the state of looking good and feeling good, we in the fitness industry have to find ways to take the fear out of exercise. The images of perfection and athleticism in fitness have to go. These images have become prevalent in our society because extremes attract attention. It's not newsworthy to show a picture of a hundred women who each have two children and who are all within 10 percent of their ideal body weights, comfortable with themselves, and looking fine. The most overweight person in the world will get in the news. Images of the fittest, most toned body in the world will have people saying, "Wow, look at that."

Magazines and TV make money from portraying extreme imperfection or extreme perfection. They will tell you there are a thousand different ways to strengthen your biceps. It's not that complicated! It's the same thing as telling you there are a thousand ways to turn the steering wheel of your car. Once you do it, it's really easy. You don't need to know a thousand different ways; you only need to know one or two. Fitness is the same. The most complicated pieces of equipment in a gym are barbells and dumbbells. You don't need to use them. Most of the consumer magazines emphasize them, but you never have to touch one. If you do decide to use the weights, someone can teach you in six easy sessions.

Even fitness classes are designed so anyone can just do them. There are advanced classes that are more complicated, but you don't need to go to them to get fit. People go for the challenge. You'll get fit whether or not you take up the challenge of higher-skill classes. It's also true that some people will join a fitness club, start becoming fit, and then discover they have some athletic talent. So they run marathons, perfect their golf games, or win squash games. That's not everybody, and it doesn't have to be you.

If the statistics continue to indicate that 75 to 85 percent of people don't participate in exercise, I can foresee that our longevity as a nation may decrease by a couple of years. We'll begin to pay the price for our lack of activity. On the other hand, if we can move from 17 to 30 percent of the population participating in exercise to 40 percent, that will create an enormous jump in positive health outcomes.

If things continue as they are now, a huge gap is going to form between overweight people dying younger, with a greater cost to the health and social systems, and the people who are carrying those costs and getting mad about it. There is a backlash now against smokers. They have more sick days, are less productive, and die sooner, and, in the process of dying, they cost the health system more. Non-smokers now outnumber smokers, and there is mounting pressure to combat nicotine addiction further. Ten or 30 years down the road we may see the same backlash against lazy, inactive people.

Let's get back to feeling good. What other things can we say about feeling good through fitness? Even sex is better if you're fit. Your body looks better. It turns your partner on more. You feel better to touch. You have the physical capability to last longer and enjoy yourself. You're not going to have a heart attack or pull a muscle in the process. It's fun. It feels good.

Exercise also has positive effects on depression. It is a powerful antidepressant. Studies have shown that exercise elevates mood. A lot of emotional problems are caused by feelings of loss of control. If you feel in control, you feel better about yourself. The first step toward gaining control is doing what you innately know is right—physical activity.

Feeling good is an intangible that, paradoxically, is tangible. It's hard to describe in exact words, but you know it when you feel it. You can't bottle it. You can't save it. You can't store it. It's like a smile—it's just there.

SOME OF OUR
CLUB MEMBERS
ON FEELING GOOD

JEFF D.

I HAD TOTALLY given up on ever being in shape. When I got on the scale and saw that number, 339 pounds, I believed it was impossible to lose it. I was wrong.

I was at work one day and started feeling terrible. I was having chest pain, having trouble breathing, and I was scared. I was taken to the hospital, and the whole time I was thinking that at my age I was having a heart attack. Luckily, I was wrong again.

That day scared my girlfriend enough that she decided to get me help. The next day I was in the gym. Since I started working out, I've felt great. When you walk in the door you can feel this great sense of community. It feels like a family there, everyone pushing each other, everyone feeling connected by mutual goals. Working with my trainer has been incredible. He pushes me to work harder than I ever have! He is always challenging me, always takes time to answer any questions, goes over every step of the exercise, and helps with meal planning and food choices.

Today I'm proud to say I've gone from 339 pounds to 181 pounds—I've lost over 150 pounds! I am just six pounds away from my goal, and I have never felt better.

I look at life in a whole new light. I don't see things I can't do anymore. I just see challenges to overcome. I am looking forward to hitting my goal weight before my wedding to the most amazing woman in this world, the one who started me on this journey. I can never thank her enough for that.

My family has told me that, through my story, people they know have been inspired and have been getting in shape. That's truly a great feeling. If we can do it, so can you!

LYNNE M.

I WOKE UP one day, after a few hectic years of raising three young sons, to find I had a low energy level, poor sleeping patterns, falling self-esteem because my clothes were not fitting the way I swore they did the week before, and increased irritability from coping with a full-time job and a growing, active family.

I had faithfully worked out with weights and performed cardiovascular activities three times a week for years. However, I had fallen into the trap of not challenging myself and trying new things. I was determined to see changes in my body composition and cardiovascular endurance and, in turn, see positive changes to my general appearance, self-esteem, stress-coping abilities, and eating habits.

With the assistance and encouragement of GoodLife staff and a personal trainer, my lifestyle changed dramatically. My experience has given me a better understanding of the importance of resistance training with cardiovascular activity, increased awareness of how food fuels your body, and a reminder of the importance of goal-setting and just plain having fun.

My body fat decreased considerably. I had copious amounts of energy, to the point that my kids could not keep up with me. I also had coworkers comment that I was much calmer and more relaxed in dealing with daily issues.

I've reached all my original goals and continue to set new, challenging ones. A desire to inform others of the benefits of physical activity, resistance training, and well-balanced eating habits led me to become certified as a personal trainer. I love this part of my life—I don't consider it work!

MARGIE M.

I AM 72, and I am sure that going to a fitness club keeps me young, healthy, and fit. I have lost inches and pounds, and I have gained many new friends. All my life I have enjoyed all sorts of sports—swimming, rowing, biking, and aerobics. So when my friends say, "At our age, we don't need it anymore," I answer, "At our age we need it twice as much." My bone density test said I have the bones of a young adult. Doing the weight training keeps them strong. I feel wonderful.

CHAPTER FIVE

A GOOD WEIGHT

EVERYONE TALKS ABOUT having a "perfect weight." We're obsessed with weight in our culture because we have tied it to our sense of selfhood and self-esteem. People will go to great lengths to "do something" about their weight. What do people mean when they say they want the perfect weight? They mean that, when they walk down the street, people will stop to cast admiring glances their way; that every photographer in the world will want to put them on the covers of fashion and lifestyle magazines; that every one of their friends will be jealous and wish they could look like them.

Wait a second. That's never going to happen for you. You will never make yourself happy with someone else's opinion of what your weight should be. All those criteria of weight I've just mentioned are based on someone else's opinion. You need to decide what your weight should be, a weight that takes into account your body type and lifestyle, the weight that will make you happy.

When it comes to weight, the influence of public media is insidious. Several times in this book you will find me saying that we must be wary of the images of perfection we see in magazines, on TV, and in the movies. Ninety-nine percent of the population simply cannot look like those models and celebrities. In fact, very often when you see a model or movie star in person, you find he or she doesn't look nearly so perfect in the flesh as on the page or the screen.

Oftentimes we find ourselves buying into the obsession with perpetual thinness, which is the current cultural ideal, often with very negative results for our health and self-esteem. We lose sight of the fact that different periods of history have had differing images of attractiveness. Some eras have valued the full-figured body, just as our era seems to be going to extremes with thinness. We need to learn to distinguish between a good weight, which is possible for us, and a perfect weight, which doesn't exist. We need to know the difference between a good weight and overweight. We need to understand that our body weight is an aspect of our overall health and that our ideal weight is the weight we are when our bodies are functioning at their best.

WHAT IS A
GOOD WEIGHT?

THE RIGHT WEIGHT for you as an individual depends on a number of factors. First of all, take into consideration your role in life. Are you a competitive athlete? Competitive athletes make up only a small percentage of the total population. Let's assume that only 2 percent of people could be classified as such. They need to have lower body fat so they can move faster. If you are one of them, you're likely training regularly and understand your diet patterns well enough that body weight is not an issue. Most athletes will have a good weight that is determined by their sport, how they train, and how they compete.

Many more people in the population are recreational athletes, taking up sports for fun and pleasure, and maybe mild competition as well. In this group, a man's body weight should be 10 to 20 percent fat, and a woman's should be between 15 and 25 percent fat, depending on whether they are ectomorphs, endomorphs, or mesomorphs. These body-fat percentages are good guidelines, even if you're not a recreational athlete.

Most people are not athletes, recreational or otherwise. In fact, as I've been saying, the pursuit of fitness is something quite separate from athleticism. So let's look at body fat in the average population. There are many methods of estimating body fat and body fat distribution these days. Suffice it to say that the World Health Organization considers people to be obese if they have a body mass index (calculation using weight and height) of 30 or more. This is unhealthy—it's going to reduce how long you live, and it's going to cut down on the quality of your life every single day.

Rather than reading charts that say if you're such and such a height, your weight should be *x*, it's far better to use body-fat percentage as your guideline. No matter what your height or your bone structure, if the percentage of total body fat falls within an acceptable range, you will be a good weight. If you are a man, and you have 10 to 15 percent body fat, you should be happy with that. That's a really good weight. You wouldn't want to weigh less than that, and there's no need to. If you are a woman, and you have around 20 to 25 percent body fat, that's a good weight for most women. You should be within these parameters of body fat, between 10 and 30 percent, which is a pretty flexible range that allows for all kinds of body types. In reality, for most people, it's between 15 and 25 percent.

I would tell a man that if he reaches 20 percent body fat, he should be thinking about increasing exercise and decreasing his intake of calories—now, before it gets ahead of him. I would say the same to a woman who reaches 30 percent body fat.

The point is, whether you're male or female, if you weigh 150 pounds and 29 percent of your weight is body fat, you are overweight. But if you weigh 200 pounds and 15 percent of your weight is body fat, you are not overweight. The variation between 10 and 30 percent takes into account your body type (ectomorph, endomorph, or mesomorph), whether you're male or female, the age and stage of life you are at, the stress level you might be experiencing, whether you're competitive or more laid-back, how active you are, and so forth. Once you drop below 10 percent body fat, you are underfed (unless you are a high-level athlete). You're not getting enough nutrition. This condition affects only a small percentage of the population. By far, the majority of us are overfed.

Body fat can be measured with fat calipers or with bio-impedance testing (a form of body composition analysis). These methods can measure how much water is in your body, how much bone, how much muscle, and so forth. A well-trained and qualified fitness professional can help you determine the ratio of body fat in your overall weight.

The tests take only about five or ten minutes. The feedback from the tests takes longer than the actual tests because most of us are distressed at first to discover that we're carrying too much body fat. This is the starting point from which you can begin to make healthy decisions to do something about your excess fat. Even if you don't take fat-measurement tests, your mirror is a good gauge. If you look at your naked body in the mirror and there are two or three inches of fat hanging over your waist, it's likely that you have too much body fat.

If you want to make it even simpler, you should be concerned about your weight if much more than three centimetres or one inch hangs over your belt or waistband when you are standing.

FACTOR IN
EATING

EXERCISE PLAYS A crucial role in weight control, but eating patterns factor in, as well. It's possible to be fit and fat. You can exercise like crazy and still be eating way too much. For example, when I ran the Boston Marathon, I weighed 225 pounds. During the years that I rowed, I weighed between 200 and 210. I rowed four hours a day, which is not something most of the population would do. However, when I ran, it was only three times a week. I ran hard and long so my body would adjust to running the distance. I also ate way too much. In the process of training for the marathon, I gained 15 pounds. It's not just how much you eat, it's also the quality of your food. Eating protein, complex carbohydrates, fruits, and vegetables makes infinitely more sense than ingesting fats, such as greasy French fries. We all know this—we so easily "forget."

Sometimes we may think a person is at a good weight, but his or her appearance is deceiving. Some people look really slim but are tremendously unfit and weak. All they're doing is not eating. Other people have phenomenally low metabolisms and have trouble losing any weight at all, no matter what they do in terms of nutrition. Still others have high metabolisms and have trouble keeping weight on. People with extremely low and high metabolisms often need professional help to help them adjust their weight in a positive direction.

The majority of us are somewhere in the middle: normal metabolisms, eating too much, but not enough of the right foods, and not getting enough exercise. We all want to know what a good weight is for us and how to get there. You know when you feel good. Your body knows when it feels healthy and vital. You look in the mirror, and you see a body that's healthy and functioning well and looks good both in and out

SOME OF MY FAVOURITE FOODS

- I eat gluten-free foods because of my arthritis.
- I don't drink coffee, but I love organic chocolate milk and green tea.
- I eat some red meat but mainly consume fresh fish.
- I eat Caesar salad without the croutons, but I triple the garlic.
- I love anything chocolate. I call chocolate my fifth main food group. It's my motivator and reward.
- I love peanut butter, especially on a cinnamon bagel.
- I love squash, turnips, and sweet potatoes.
- My favourite fruit is pineapple.
- I tried being a vegetarian once, but it didn't work for me.
- My favourite meal of all: my mother's hamburgers!

of clothes. If that's what you see, chances are you're the right weight for you. You can achieve 95 percent of what you want for your weight simply by participating in the type of fitness routine I have been talking about in this book—three times a week, for 20 to 30 minutes.

Wanting to lose weight is the reason most people start exercising. Exercise will help you lose weight, but it doesn't happen overnight. This is a very important point, for most of us want instant results. At first when you start exercising, you will most likely put weight on, because in the first month or two you will gain three to four pounds of muscle. Muscle weighs more than fat for the area it takes up. A 130-pound woman may say after four weeks of exercise, "Look, I've put on four pounds and now weigh 134. What's going on?" That's when I would say to her, "Don't your sweaters and pants fit looser? Don't you feel more toned? Don't you have more energy? Don't you feel good about yourself?"

It's good to take your waist, chest, and thigh measurements when you want to lose weight and stay motivated. The initial weight gain in muscle will eventually translate into an overall reduction of body fat. As you lose the body fat and replace it with muscle, your weight will gradually adjust to where it should be for you to have a healthy, vital, and good-looking body. Trust the process and be patient. It works. I never encourage people to modify their weights by not eating or by restricting their diets only. If you want to achieve weight control, you need a process of strength training and exercise combined with sensible eating. If you are simply not eating, you won't be getting enough vitamins and other nutrients. You will be on a constant seesaw between how much you eat versus how you look, and you will never be happy. Be patient with yourself. You can do this!

WHY DIETING DOESN'T WORK

DIETING IS A way of training your body to cope with starvation mode. When you restrict your caloric intake to below what your body needs to feel satisfied, your body responds as it would have five thousand years ago, when maybe the crops had failed or the hunters came back empty-handed. When the body senses starvation, it stores as much fat as it can. Evolutionary biology has trained us to do that very efficiently.

At the same time, if you starve the body, the body will break down muscles in order to get protein and energy, and as a result you get weaker. Remember that every pound of muscle uses 50 to 100 calories a day. When you break down a pound of muscle in the course of dieting, you will look as if you're losing weight. You won't understand why your body doesn't look that much better and why you don't feel that much better. It's the opposite when you start exercising. Initially you put on some weight, but it's muscle. In the long run, exercise will help you lose fat and keep it off, and in the short run, you'll look and feel better.

If you go off the diet where you lost muscle from starvation dieting and begin eating as much as you used to, you'll quickly start to gain weight again. In addition, because you don't have the muscle you had before, you'll put weight on faster than you did before you dieted.

When you're on a diet that gives you fewer calories than you need, your body reacts as though it's threatened with starvation. So it will do what it knows it should do: it will push you to eat. That's why you crave food when you're on a diet, feel an increase in appetite, and fall off the wagon. You have to be superhuman to control your hunger.

A further problem is that our bodies also assume that we will engage in physical activity to build muscle back up, because for thousands of years that's exactly what we did. In the last 50 years, our society has become increasingly sedentary. In the past, we had to plant crops, run across fields, lift logs to make our houses, and battle the elements. Today we can just go back to our computer terminals or turn on the TV. Our bodies don't put on muscle from day-to-day living anymore. So if you've lost weight by dieting, or if you've been sick, you should work with weights, either through circuit training, team training, or a group exercise class, to build up your strength. It's the only way to rebuild muscle. The way to really lose weight and keep it off is to combine strength training while controlling your eating patterns.

CONTROLLING
YOUR EATING

THERE IS A difference between dieting and controlling your eating. Dieting is just an across-the-board reduction of the number of calories you take in, often without regard for your body type, lifestyle, or activity level. Controlling your eating, on the other hand, involves saying to yourself something like, "For normal function, I need three thousand calories. I need these calories from different types of food: for example, a third from protein, a third from carbohydrates, and a third from fruits and vegetables." This is very different from just cutting back.

Humans are omnivores. We need a balance of different types of food. Even vegetarian animals consume different types of plants. The majority of species survive by having variety in their diets. The coyote, which can survive in literally all environments, including cities and towns, will eat anything.

Controlling your eating means taking in the calories you need through the right balance of nutrition from the different food groups. It means making wise choices: for example, choosing a baked potato over French fries, or oil-and-vinegar dressing on your salad over creamy ranch dressing. Generally, a woman needs about 2,500 calories a day, and a man 3,500.

There are some variations, depending on your age, size, and level of activity. There are very few people who can satisfy their bodies' natural hunger with fewer than a thousand calories per day. So if you go on a diet of a thousand calories or less, you know you're getting less than half the normal intake you need. You're going to lose a lot of muscle. Furthermore, the body will take those thousand calories and convert them to fat. It will break down your biceps, quadriceps, and back muscles in order to get energy.

You're going to get a much more desirable result, however, by controlling your eating patterns within the proper number of calories for your lifestyle and body type and strength training. If you control your eating patterns but don't strength train, up to 80 percent of what you eventually lose will be muscle. If you do strength train, almost everything you burn off will be fat, and the food you take in will be used to build muscle. The key to a good weight is to eat within your normal caloric range and to exercise, incorporating strength training into your routine.

One of the misconceptions about exercise and weight control is that you need to do a lot of cardiovascular training to burn calories. You need cardiovascular exercise to improve your heart and lungs, to get your whole "pipe system" working better. However, this type of exercise burns calories while you're exercising. You also need exercises that build muscle, because muscles burn calories all the time. By adding muscle, you don't have to eat less to burn off the calories. If you miss a week of cardiovascular training, you'll lose 10 percent of your cardiovascular efficiency. If you build muscle over six months, it will take that long to lose it should you stop exercising. If, for some reason, you miss some strength training—for example, if you're ill or on vacation—you have more of a "cushion" of strength. You will be able to regain strength quite readily when you restart the exercises.

To me, achieving a good weight is not about denying yourself food. It's about balance. In fact, weight control shouldn't be painful. It should include enough leeway to allow occasional indulgence in your pet "not good for you" food group. In my case, that's chocolate. For some, it might be a cold beer, or a hamburger with all the trimmings. You should never see achieving a good weight as a path of deprivation. It doesn't have to be. You can design your weight-control program to allow for a few perks.

Many people seek out professional weight-control programs from companies that claim to guarantee a certain level of weight loss within a certain length of time. Any weight-control group or program that doesn't encourage exercise is not telling the whole story. Any weight-control program that encourages extremes of caloric reduction, or that advocates ingesting great amounts of one particular food (for example, bananas or pineapples) to the exclusion of others, should be avoided. Any weight-control group that encourages exercise, along with a balanced diet, and that doesn't encourage extremes is OK. I think the best of these programs are those that teach us to make healthy choices so we can continue on our own.

EXERCISE INFLUENCES APPETITE

EXERCISE WILL HELP balance appetite for most people. It may act as an appetite suppressant for some, but this is rare and even for them is not consistent. I think the most far-reaching effect of exercise on appetite lies in the psychological aspects of our makeup. A lot of us eat as a way to cope with stress. As children we learned that when we fell down and hurt ourselves, Mom would give us candy or a cookie to help us feel better. The idea was ingrained in many of us that eating makes us feel better emotionally. Often exercise will control the urge to eat because of its positive effect on stress levels. Exercise helps us feel less stress so, by extension, it reduces the artificially created need to eat so as not to feel sad or stressed out.

Exercise also stabilizes blood sugar levels and in this way helps you avoid the ups and downs of blood sugar that may cause you to want to eat. Then there is what I call the ripple effect of exercising on eating. You decide to exercise. You do it, and it feels good. In the back of your mind is the thought, "I have just exercised. I need to be a little smarter about what I eat." The self-control you achieve through exercise extends to other areas of your life and gives you the resolve you need to carry through with healthy lifestyle decisions.

Exercise and proper nutrition together help your body become a self-regulating system that will find its own wisdom for health within. Exercise and good nutrition support how your body is designed to work. Something that's running the way it's supposed to likes to stay that way. When you see a horse galloping in the pasture, you can tell that it loves to run. You just know. You don't need to prove it—you can see it in the flex and stretch of its sleek muscles and the speed and grace of its movements. It's the same for people. When you exercise and it feels good, and when you eat healthfully and it feels good, you know that it feels good, that it's right.

Trust your body to tell you what's good. All you have to do is listen. We're really good at hearing the negative messages from our bodies, but not so good at paying attention to the positive ones. For example, if you bang your leg on a table and get a bruise, your body will register "ouch," and you will think, "This is bad. This is distressing." Think of it the other way around. You're exercising and eating well and your body sends you signals that say, "My blood is circulating freely. My skin looks better. I have more energy. It's easier to stand straight. I find things aren't bugging me as much. My stress level is lower." These signals are telling you that you're doing what you're supposed to do.

If you pay attention to your body, eventually you'll know instinctively how much food you need and how much activity your body needs. In this culture, we have to relearn these instincts because we've lost touch with the intuitive health wisdom within us. That's why I think personal trainers and well-trained nutrition and exercise experts are so helpful. They understand the need for balance and avoiding extremes. Ultimately, though, you can become your own expert. Give your body what it needs in terms of physical activity and balanced nutrition, and you will be rewarded with a good weight that you'll find easy to maintain. You'll wake up every morning happy with the way you are.

SOME OF OUR
CLUB MEMBERS
ON A GOOD WEIGHT

CASSANDRA D.

MY ENTIRE LIFE has been a struggle with obesity. Even as a young child I can remember being self-conscious and embarrassed by my weight. As I grew older, the problems escalated. I tried all the fad diets without success and eventually resigned myself to being fat forever. In 1997, my weight reached an all-time high of 290 pounds. As a registered nurse, I understood the consequences of my excessive weight and feared for my health. Day-to-day activities had become a struggle. I became short of breath with minimal exertion, and my legs and hips ached constantly. I worried continuously about things most people take for granted: would I be able to find clothes that fit me? Would I fit into the seat at the theatre? Were people laughing at me? I felt like my entire life was out of control.

Finally, several years ago, I faced a health crisis that made me realize that I had to take control of my weight. I joined GoodLife Fitness the next day, and my life has changed completely.

The trainers at the gym immediately put me at ease and made me realize that I was not alone in my battle of the bulge. Every six weeks, I met with a personal trainer who helped me design an exercise program specific to my needs. Within weeks, I began to see results. The pounds started to drop, and I noticed a slow but steady increase in my energy level and stamina. As the months progressed, I was literally able to watch my body transform. Muscle replaced fat, and my entire appearance began to change. I was elated each time I was able to move down a dress size. The regular program checks motivated me to stay on track and push myself a little harder. And on the occasions when my spirits lagged or I felt defeated, there was always someone there to address my concerns and get me back on track. Within a year, I was less than 10 pounds away from my target weight of 160 pounds. Finally, I reached my goal!

I continued to set new goals, and exercise is now an integral part of my life. I feel that my weight is now under my control, rather than in control of me. I am healthier and happier than I have ever been, and I am no longer ashamed and embarrassed by my body.

Since my weight loss, I enjoy a much more active lifestyle. The increase in my level of confidence and self-esteem has helped me to form many new and healthy relationships. I even credit GoodLife with giving me the emotional wellbeing that led me to the man I am about to marry. Despite the occasional setback, I know that I will never go back to the unhealthy lifestyle I once lived.

DAVID T.

BY BECOMING INVOLVED with fitness, I was able to achieve goals that had eluded me for years. Like most people, I had put on some undesirable weight over the years, and my blood pressure was up a little. I had tried a variety of programs to lose the weight, but nothing really worked. Using the GoodLife method, I was able to lose weight, increase my muscle strength, and lower my blood pressure.

I saw an advertisement for a personal training program at the club and decided to give it a try. I lost the weight I wanted to lose. In particular, as the fat was lost, my clothes became noticeably looser. My waist size went down to a level it had not been in 20 years.

I was able to fit the program easily into my lifestyle. Because the workouts were brief, I could do them during my lunch hour. The training was challenging but not beyond my capabilities. In addition, I found the diet plan excellent. The food I was required to eat was very similar to what I usually ate. By spreading meals out into many smaller portions during the day, I found I was not always hungry, and was able to adhere to my training. I found the suggested recipes to be very tasty, and I have continued to use many of them in my current eating patterns.

I wanted to lose some additional weight after the program was completed. To do this, I hired a personal trainer and continued with my exercise/diet plan. After 10 weeks of training and following the diet, my clothes were really loose.

I had achieved the weight I had set as a goal. The amount of fat I had lost was around 14 kilograms and I had gained 3 kilograms of muscle. In order for my clothes to fit properly, I had them altered. Although I had not been terribly overweight, my blood pressure was higher (135/85 was common) than it was in my later twenties (117/75). After I lost the weight, my blood pressure went back to the value it used to be.

I am continuing to train regularly, and my strength is steadily increasing. Strength training is not time-consuming to do, since only one set of each exercise is done to success. It is very effective in increasing strength. As a result of using interval training for the cardiovascular part of the workout and then moving quickly through the weight-training section, my cardiovascular fitness has improved and my heart rate has lowered.

CHAPTER SIX

A GOOD RECOVERY

BOOKS ON FITNESS often focus on people who are "normally healthy" and don't take into account the fact that life sometimes deals us a tough hand. There will be times when we're altogether healthy, and other times when we're faced with a chronic health condition or traumatic event.

Can fitness play a role in recovery from accidents and illness? Can it help people who have a chronic condition achieve a higher quality of life?

My answer to those questions is a resounding yes. I know this from my own experience and from the experiences of GoodLife members who have used fitness to aid in their recoveries or to help them cope with health conditions.

MY
MOTORCYCLE
ACCIDENT

EARLIER I TALKED a bit about the serious motorcycle accident
I had when I was starting university. The accident was life
changing for me, for it brought me into a career of helping
people pursue fitness.

I was going too fast, as is usual for almost anyone who
rides a motorcycle. A car signalled left but turned right . . .
whack! I didn't want to go through the car's windshield, so
I held on as hard as I could to the bike's handlebars. As a
result, I flipped up and over, my heels hit the roof of the car,
I landed on the grass, and the motorcycle landed on me.
With a superhuman burst of adrenalin-pumped strength, I
threw the 400-pound bike off me to about four feet away.
Then I couldn't move—not my head, my fingers, my legs—
nothing. Things were going in slow motion in my head, and
pain shot through me.

When an ambulance arrived, the paramedics asked me
if I could move. I remember thinking, "This is serious." As
the sensation gradually came back into my body and I could
begin to move my neck and arms, the pain became intense.
My whole body was wracked with it. The paramedics put me
on a spinal board and took me to the hospital. Four doctors

had to pull my shoulders back into alignment. There were a lot of torn cartilages, ligaments, and tendons, and my right shoulder was sitting four inches lower than my left. This began my introduction to the world of serious injuries.

Not that I had been injury-free. In my 20 short years I had managed to break feet, arms, legs, fingers, wrist, jaw, ribs, and nose. These breaks were the results of various athletic injuries, stupid injuries, "being where you shouldn't be" injuries, and risk-oriented injuries. But the motorcycle accident was really bad, because it involved multiple disabling injuries.

I spent a long time in bed convalescing. Then I was introduced to the athletic injuries clinic at Western University. As I learned to use ice and was taken through all kinds of exercising and stretching, I spent a lot of time talking to other patients and their therapists.

I became interested in how the healing process works. How do you get better after an injury? What drives you to recover and become strong again? The healing process is different for every joint in the body, but general practices do apply: rest, care, stretching, and the overload principle of exercise, "making it stronger faster." You have to apply yourself constantly. The sooner you can make yourself do a movement, the better for your recovery.

I asked myself, "Why does one person get better faster than another?" Is one stretch better than another stretch? How much depends on the head, on what you're thinking? How much depends on the body? I began to realize that a crucial component of recovery is attitude. A serious injury is a major wake-up call for people who have always taken their strength and health for granted.

Looking back on that time, I can now say that my recovery actually made my body better. It forced me to think everything through. It made me learn how every muscle group worked. It showed me how hard some people will work to regain what they've lost, while others seem to give up and become apathetic.

My accident created the life I have today. At the time, as I've mentioned, I was planning to go to the business school at the university. I might even have become a banker. It was my accident that got me thinking about the value of getting the body to be the best it can be. My goal, to recover my physical strength and to emerge mentally stronger, ultimately led me to my career.

When I looked at fitness clubs at the time, I saw that what they had in common was doing sales. They sold memberships and used all kinds of enticements to get people to buy. None of them really understood fitness. The people who did understand fitness—for example, the kinesiologists and exercise physiologists at the university—didn't know how to sell people on fitness or how to motivate people. When I say sell, I mean they didn't know how to encourage them, motivate them, make them want to participate, make them buy in to the fact that they're wonderful and they can do it—in other words, to sell people on their own potential. I became consumed by the question of how to make people be the best they can be—to help them play a better squash game; to make them stand straighter, get stronger, go faster; to train their hearts and lungs; to help them gain maximum flexibility.

Later, that following autumn, I began rowing. Rowing is a continuous, rhythmic action. It gets under your skin and feels really good, but it's hard work. To do it, you have to be very fit. You have to be strong, both muscularly and psychologically. You need good flexibility, phenomenal muscular endurance, and a great heart and lungs. Because of all these different aspects, you have to learn what parts of the body to focus on training during which part of the year and then focus on training other parts later. You have to learn about training cycles. You have to learn how to go faster, as an individual and as a team, without getting injured. An athlete always operates on that fine edge between exhaustion and exhilaration. Many people go through life like that. They're almost exhausted, and they're almost at the peak of their power. For general fitness, you don't have to be that close to the edge.

It was the motorcycle accident and my subsequent experiences as a competitive athlete that led me to the business I am in now. The recovery from the accident, and my status as a high-level athlete who had won five Canadian rowing championships, gave me credibility and also helped me understand something very crucial: what it's like to be on the edge of both very good and exhausted. From that I learned that fitness can indeed be used to push us to recovery from injuries and accidents.

AN INJURY CAN BE AN OPPORTUNITY

OFTEN WHEN PEOPLE have an automobile accident or some other kind of serious accident, they're forced to slow down and focus on their bodies. All of a sudden they become in tune with a body they've been ignoring or have taken for granted all those years. Some become resentful that their body couldn't hold up against two tons of steel. Some think the injuries are just going to heal by themselves. That doesn't happen. Major injuries require good rehabilitation. As they go through the rehabilitation process, many people begin to think, "Hey, this is pretty miraculous what I have here—my body's capacity to heal, its capacity to function—and I'm going to get that back, or at least get back the best quality of life I can."

Many people who give it a shot are really amazed at how fast their body can recover, and they're surprised by how fast their mental outlook improves, too. They experience, often for the first time, the pleasure of doing something really physical. For some people, the experience of doing rehabilitation exercises for half an hour every day leads them to establish a lifelong habit of fitness. I've known many people for whom an injury ended up making their life better. Think of an injury as an opportunity to discover more about yourself. It's a chance for you to think of alternatives, try something different, and change your mindset.

Anybody who does any active sport runs the risk of injury. With our increased longevity, most of us will have some kind of injury at some point. If you're actively involved in fitness at a club, there's a low chance you're going to injure yourself. If you don't do anything active, you also risk injury, because you've become weak and susceptible. Back problems, for example, are epidemic in this society. Some 80 to 90 percent of back problems are caused by weak muscles. Injuries happen when muscles get weak. If you work on your back, on getting your heart stronger, and on strengthening your shoulders and knees, you'll be able to prevent many nasty, weakness-induced injuries. You're far more likely to get injured if you're unfit.

I think doctors are cautious when it comes to a person's recovery capabilities. When they're treating a condition, their clinical diagnoses may be based on what has worked in the past. For an injury, and for many other conditions, doctors cannot categorically predict the course of recovery. They often don't want to raise what they think may be false expectations.

A lot of people think they are owed a healthy body, or perfect healing from an injury, especially if the injury wasn't their fault. For example, if the car that hit theirs went through a red light, or their injury at work was the result of inadequate safety mechanisms, they may become consumed with anger and resentment and have a sense of entitlement about recovery. The concept of entitlement robs you of your freedom, because you are laying your happiness in someone else's lap. You think you can't be happy unless you get x dollars in compensation or x amount of care. What you have to realize is that happiness is a personal choice about taking control of your own life, and that your recovery is, within the limits of the injury, in your hands.

Many people ask me about injuries in fitness clubs. Overall, fitness clubs have a very low rate of injuries. You can get an injury from overtraining, which tends to happen to athletes. You can get an injury from failing to do something right. Most clubs have easy-to-use, standardized equipment and qualified people to show you how. The equipment, if it is good, is designed to do it right. When people follow the right procedures and get the right guidance, injuries in fitness clubs are few and far between.

FITNESS AND CHRONIC CONDITIONS

LET'S SAY YOU have a shoulder that always hurts. You need to do two things. One is to exercise your whole body to reduce the stress on that particular shoulder and what it has to do. The second is to exercise the shoulder so everything you give it becomes a bit easier. Your body always fails at its weakest link. Your job, then, is simply to make your weakest link as strong as it can be.

For many of us, our weakest link takes the form of some kind of chronic condition: arthritis, diabetes, chronic fatigue syndrome, heart disease, asthma. A chronic condition is different from an injury. With an injury, you hope for recovery. This can keep you motivated in your exercise rehabilitation. But with a chronic condition, there is no "recovery." There is no pot of gold at the end of the rainbow. There is only "the problem." You can decide whether this can be a good problem. Often the first thing that happens when you get diagnosed with a chronic disease is denial. The second phase is self-pity: "Why me?" The third phase is the choice between giving in or fighting.

When I was diagnosed with rheumatoid arthritis at 32, my entire body was filled with pain. My hands and feet wouldn't work. I could barely move. All this had hit me out of the blue the day after I had won a rowing championship. Overnight I went from high-level racer to invalid. At first I thought I had an athletics-induced arthritis that I had brought on myself by pushing the limits. It never occurred to me that it could be rheumatoid arthritis, even though that condition runs in my family. It didn't occur to my doctors at first, either.

When the diagnosis was confirmed, the doctors told me not to exercise. I obeyed them for a few weeks, but found I was just getting weaker. In my usual headstrong manner, I decided to go ahead and exercise, just as I had always told everyone else to do. When I got back onto a stationary bicycle, I had to have someone help me turn the wheels. After about six weeks, I could turn the wheels myself. Then they had to help me with the weights, after which everything hurt. But gradually I began to notice an improvement.

With any chronic illness, you need to figure out how to be as strong as you can be, all over. I knew this from my background in exercise physiology. If you can put up with the pain from the exercise, you'll feel better later. At first I had arthritis attacks every three months that lasted four to six weeks. Then the attack frequency went to every four months, then every six months, and it is continuing to decrease. Not only have the attacks lessened, but continuing to build up my strength continues to serve me well when I do get an attack.

The same endorphins that make the average, healthy person feel good during and after exercise will help people who are exercising to manage the pain or discomfort of a chronic illness.

When I was 36 I decided to get into downhill skiing. Because of the arthritis, I couldn't use my shoulders to get up out of the snow. I couldn't hold onto the poles or push on them. When I fell, I got up by collecting my legs under me and rolling over onto my back. Then I crossed my arms on my chest and used my thigh muscles to raise myself up. There was no way I was going to allow arthritis to keep me from skiing. There are people who ski with only one limb, or without any legs at all, or even blind. Now that's courage!

The older you get, the more likely it is that you will have a chronic condition to deal with. As we age, we need to learn how to deal with these conditions. I consider that my arthritis made my business successful. It made me a happier, more caring person. It helped me not to take things for granted. When you can't even open a car door for yourself and you have to wait for people to do things for you, you begin to understand some of the problems that other people may have. If you have a chronic condition and you improve the quality of your life by managing it well, your value for life increases. Even though I may be strong enough today to go outside and smell the flowers or see the stars, I wake up every morning knowing that I might not be able to do that tomorrow. Having arthritis has made me highly empathetic. When someone comes into a GoodLife club and says, "I've never been able to work out," or "I was always laughed at in high school," or "I'm too old and out of shape, and I don't feel well," I know what that person is feeling.

Many chronic conditions, such as diabetes, arthritis, or chronic fatigue, are insidious—you can't see them. These conditions, though, can be turned around to actually become life enhancing based on how you choose to react to them. Maybe their onset shocks you into taking care of yourself. Taking care, taking control, doing something—all give you good hope. In the fitness industry, more and more we find we are working with people who have chronic conditions. The baby boomer generation forms a large part of fitness clubs' clientele, and, as the boomers grow older, they will be confronting their mortality and the physical conditions that go with aging. Increasingly, fitness clubs are designing programs for older adults aimed at enhancing quality of life and achieving a good level of fitness for each person as an individual, no matter what conditions he or she may be battling.

Heart disease is the number one cause of hospitalization in Canada, affecting more than 1.3 million Canadians. Many risk factors—poor diet, sedentary lifestyle, stress—are on the rise. In 2012, seeing a unique opportunity to help, I entered into collaboration with University Health Network, a group of hospitals in the Toronto area, by funding an internationally recognized Centre of Excellence in cardiac health and exercise. The then President and CEO, Dr. Bob Bell (now Ontario's Deputy Minister of Health), was united with us in our belief in the vital importance of activity and exercise in cardiac rehabilitation. He stated, "This will foster knowledge and innovation in cardiac health, reducing readmissions of current patients and preventing cardiac episodes from the outset. This will save lives and help to reduce the cost of care in Ontario." For my part, being a contributor meant we would directly help patients and their families. We would also be one step closer to fulfilling our purpose: "to give Canadians the opportunity to live fit and healthy lives." As part of this collaboration, we spent the following two years working with cardiologists at UHN to develop a cardiac rehabilitation personal training specialization program delivered by GoodLife across Canada to help patients achieve lifelong success in their cardiac rehabilitation and health.

"Good hope" is taking what is dealt to you and turning it around. It's deciding that you can make the best of what's happening in your life. After all, you could just as easily decide to make things worse. There are people who do incredible things despite great odds. If you're even trying to improve your health and fitness, congratulate yourself and feel good, because many people are not even trying.

If you have a chronic condition, "doing fitness" is not going to cure you, but you will increase your quality of life, minimize the impact of the condition, and maximize your opportunities for health and well-being. Most people don't even know I have rheumatoid arthritis. On average, I'm stronger than most men my age, and I always want to have that edge.

There is no reason why you can't have that edge, too!

CARING FOR
TOUGH EMOTIONS

I WANT TO say something about some of the tough emotions that can affect us. We know that exercise can help you recover from injuries and will help you manage chronic conditions. However, often when we end up in the throes of some really tough emotions, we are tempted to let our self-care routines (of which exercise is one) slide. It's not just about maintaining exercise, though. If we're living a good life, this entails knowing that we are indeed going to encounter emotionally difficult situations. Let's look at a couple of these.

Very often, when people start talking about happiness, particularly about the fact that happiness can actually be a choice and that a positive attitude improves your life, optimistic people get accused of sugarcoating reality. There is a difference between having a healthy positive attitude and being blindly positive. Blind positivity is naïve. Realistic positivity is wise.

One of the inevitabilities of life is that we're going to face grief and loss at some point. Truly optimistic people do not deny or ignore the fact that bad things can and do happen. Realistic optimists do not deny that life has its ups and downs. Nor do they deny the reality of loss in our lives. We cannot go through life without losing something or someone we love. Loss is real. It's painful. It hurts. We shed tears. We feel broken. It actually causes a disturbance to our physiology. A happy life is not a life devoid of grief, loss, or disappointment. Someone we love dies, we get passed over for a promotion, we lose our job, a person we thought we could count on lets us down. At these times, the idea or feeling of happiness is the farthest thing from our minds. Sometimes, in the midst of a major loss, we feel we will never be happy again.

Grief counselors will tell you to allow yourself to feel the grief. They worry about people who gloss over grief, people who say, "Oh, everything is fine. I'm not doing too bad. I can manage." These may be noble sentiments, but if you've just suffered a major loss, chances are your real feelings are, "Everything is not fine, I'm having trouble coping, I'm not managing well. I don't even want to manage . . . I just want to crawl into a hole somewhere. I'm so tired." I want to suggest that these types of feelings are indeed part of your overall happiness. Think about this: happiness can only really exist if loss is real. That's a paradox—part of life's mysteries. Light can't exist without dark, up cannot exist without down, and happy cannot exist without sad. The ancient Chinese sages had it right when they talked about the idea of yin-yang, the constant changing between light and dark, between stimulation and balance, between tears and joy.

The bad stuff in our lives makes experiencing the good stuff all the more powerful. I lost my father when I was eight years old. I saw him die in an automobile accident right before my eyes. My family was faced with picking up the pieces of our lives and continuing on. My mother in an instant became a single mother. There were also economic stresses on top of the grieving. I was told that I would have to grow up faster and assume more responsibilities. Life was not the same.

However, something else was glimmering in our tragedy. We all became more resilient. My mother adopted the motto, "Never give up, don't you ever give up." She always believed in my dream and the potential of GoodLife Fitness. Whenever we ran into tough situations with the company, she would say to me, "Don't you ever give up." That attitude powered her life, my life, and my business's life. It was an attitude forged in a tragic loss. As I look back now at my childhood, I realize that my father's death contributed to my becoming a more compassionate person as an adult. I frequently encounter people at my clubs who tell me, "I had a heart attack, and I've had to stop work," or "My husband died, and I have to do something to get myself out of the house," or "I've just been diagnosed with insulin-dependent diabetes, and I'll have to live with this for the rest of my life." I've learned that it helps people a lot when I simply listen—when I am able to identify with their loss. If they ask my opinion, I usually come out with some version of "never give up."

Loss and grief are not easy for us to deal with, but they are an inevitable part of life. This consciousness that at any time we could encounter loss makes us savour our happiness even more. It points us toward enjoying and valuing the things and qualities that matter most to us: friendship, love, health, contentment, beauty in nature, a smile, an embrace, spending time around a fire.

How about disappointments? They are less intense experiences of loss, ones that, if we don't handle them with perspective, can leach the life out of us. Just as with big losses, if you've never been disappointed, if you've never failed, if you've never tried hard and didn't achieve what you wanted, then you will never understand happiness. If you've never fallen off your skis, you'll never know the feeling of skiing joyously down that mountain (and believe me, there isn't a skier anywhere who hasn't taken a tumble). If you've never had a setback, you'll never know what "going forward" means. We can choose to be consumed by our disappointments, or we can choose to learn from them. When you're confronted by a disappointment, you can ask yourself, "What is the positive side of this?" Maybe the friend who let you down revealed to you that he or she was not a good prospect as a friend and so you were able to get out of the relationship before you got in too deep. Maybe not getting the job you applied for leads you to an even better job down the road, one that you never knew existed.

I think the people who tell me they have never felt disappointment probably don't care deeply about anything. You can be disappointed only about something you care about. I find myself talking more with my children about this these days. I know that, as young people, they're entering a world where there will be some hard knocks. So when things don't go their way, I ask them for their perspective on it. I also ask them to identify what they're grateful for. I'll say more about the role gratitude plays in a happy life later.

So getting knocked down by life means that you can get back up again. Over the next few days, think about times in your life when you experienced a hard knock or perhaps lost a competition and how those times in some way or other, whether small or large, led you to experience, appreciate, and, most importantly, decide on happiness.

Through it all, do not neglect getting physical! I truly believe that regular physical activity can get you through tough times—not just physical events like accidents or illnesses, but emotional ones as well. Exercising, even gentle exercise or something as simple as going out for a walk, will help counteract the heaviness of tough feelings. It will help you cope with these feelings better. I'm not suggesting that exercise will completely take away difficult situations, but it can, and does, help to support you through them. If anything, see physical activity as you taking care of yourself. Exercise will give you the physical and energy reserves to get you through to a good recovery.

SOME OF OUR
CLUB MEMBERS ON
A GOOD RECOVERY

MAGGIE S.

HERE IS MY story. I hope it inspires others.

Seven years ago, I was diagnosed with rheumatoid arthritis, an inflammatory joint disease, as well as dermato-myositis, a muscle-degenerating disease. I was prescribed serious drugs to combat them. I suffered memory loss, depression, physical deterioration, and weight loss. I knew that, unless I made some drastic changes in my life, I was going to end up in a wheelchair.

I decided to turn to fitness. Working with me five to six days a week, with guidance and patience, my trainer helped me begin a slow process of rehabilitation. He took me through the basic stages of learning how to "crawl" and then how to "walk." He helped me to strengthen weakened muscles so that movements became efficient and strong. When joints weren't moving properly, he used manual therapy to correct them. He had a look at my diet and made changes to accom-modate my metabolism.

My mood and memory improved. I started to regain muscle mass. I was taught to overcome my fears and to have the confidence to lift weights that I never thought I could. Two and a half years later, I am doing 225-pound dead lifts, 135-pound squats, and 155-pound bench-presses.

I am a strong, confident 57-year-old. I am off all medications, and my diseases are in remission. I am in the best shape that I have ever been in my life!

DONALDA G.

I WISH TO tell you how fitness has changed my life for the better. The story I have to share starts out tragically but ends on a note of triumph. I am a survivor of a violent crime. Despite reconstructive surgery, I was left disabled with crippling pain. This tragedy left me not only physically broken, but the person I was inside disappeared.

I was always an outgoing and fit person, but this violation caused me to hide away in shame. I turned to food for comfort, and felt safer as my fit and healthy body gained pound after pound.

As time progressed I lost hope that I would ever be able to regain the healthy body I once had. With the love of family and friends, plus the support of doctors and therapists, I was able to regain a sense of self-worth and wholeness. However, the injuries to my body are permanent, and there is nothing more that medicine can do for me except relieve my suffering with drugs. With regret I accepted the fact that I would never be able to go for bike rides or hike a trail with my boys and husband again. The reality of the journey before me often left me feeling full of despair.

However, my life was given a new direction. As a birthday present, my husband bought me a membership to a GoodLife club. I was excited at the thought of exercising again, but at the same time I was fearful that I would injure myself or fail miserably. I couldn't comprehend how I was to travel this road alone.

Fortunately, I was not alone. From the first day I arrived at the gym, I received overwhelming support from the staff. Several of the personal trainers went out of their way to help me get a healthy body. I felt safe at the club, knowing that the trainers were there watching over me with special care. One trainer often stopped just to talk and encourage me. She listened with care as I shared my anxiety over my limitations and self-image. A class instructor took extra time, one-on-one, to help me modify the movements my body was unable to perform. It amazes me how far I have come. In a very short time, I lost 11 pounds and 17.75 millimetres of body fat. My strength improved and my physical pain became more manageable. But more important, I regained something I thought I had lost forever—the confidence to grow.

Six days a week I awake with a path set before me. Whenever I stumble, the staff are there to help me find my strength to go another mile. I probably will never win a contest or an award for physical excellence, but that is all right. You see, I'm already a winner. I've been given a second boost on the road to a good life.

JAMES C.

FROM CHILDHOOD WE are told that life holds many surprises and is full of unpredictable and sometimes life-altering events. Yet we are frequently ill-prepared to face these realities when they show up at our doors. Most of the time we can wing our way through, but once in a while nothing seems to work. So it was in the spring of 1996, at the age of 50, that I faced one of these unexpected visitors.

With a long and painful separation behind me and the reality of losing my nest egg, I took up rollerblading as a means of physically, spiritually, and symbolically getting back on track. The future appeared wide open until one day in May. While I was slaloming down a wooden bridge, the wheels of one skate dropped through a crack as my upper body rotated downhill. Sixteen weeks later, the cast was removed. I was faced with the task of rebuilding a leg and dealing with unsolicited advice about acting my age. Four months of rehab got my ankle working, but my mental edge was gone. My confidence was lacking. My goal of moving forward seemed like a distant dream. Perhaps my critics were right in telling me that a more sedentary life was more appropriate for an "aged warrior."

One visit to a fitness club convinced me to try another approach. Six weeks later, on my birthday, I stood at the top of the "Elevator Shaft" looking down through the moguls on the ski slope. I had a flashback of standing at the top of the stairs with crutches under my arms, working up the courage to take that first step. It was a new experience on a ski hill to feel the cold chill that comes with fear. Fortunately, another flashback occurred, showing me why I was here in the first place. I remember the feel of the wind stinging my face and my legs moving in slow motion to their own rhythm, winding through the bumps. Time stood still. Somehow I reached the bottom still on my feet, heart pounding and out of breath but totally pumped! It was a rush unlike anything previously experienced—and I have never looked back.

I continue to work out regularly and have picked up squash again after 10 years. As far as getting on track again, this life-enhancing experience opened the door to a new career focus and a relationship I thought was well beyond my reach. And the best part of the story is this: two years after walking into the club and taking up the challenge, I became the proud and very happy father of a little boy.

When asked why I would "start again," I smile and just say, "Because I am blessed and able to do so."

KRISTA M.

I had been physically active since high school. At age 26, I slipped on a grassy hill and hurt my ankle. At first I didn't think anything of it. I noticed, though, after a time, that my ankle was not recovering well, so I made an appointment with a physiotherapist. With a concerned look on her face, she informed me that I had a physical response known as hyperreflexia, which could indicate severe upper neurological damage, often the result of a past trauma.

I thought of a car accident I had experienced a few years prior. Initially the doctors thought I had broken my neck but eventually gave me the all-clear. Several years later, when puzzling symptoms persisted, I began a difficult journey through the health care system. At first medical professionals thought I had a brain tumour, or perhaps multiple sclerosis—both were eventually ruled out. They finally diagnosed me with a condition known as Arnold-Chiari malformation. The characteristics of this condition involved my cerebellum growing into my neck and crushing some of the nerves in my spinal column. An MRI also indicated a lesion in the spinal column, and the doctors wanted to do brain surgery.

Throughout all this, I continued to work out. As the time for surgery approached, I realized that my right side was weaker than my left, and I could no longer run. The surgeons did repair the malformation and told me I wouldn't deteriorate further. However, my current condition would become the "new normal" that I would have to manage. I went back to the fitness club where the staff were supportive and welcoming. I never felt judged or uncomfortable.

On the days that were really hard—when my neck pain was almost debilitating and my workouts were not very good—I always remembered Patch's words, "Good enough is good enough." I spent the next two years having MRIs and spinal taps, and at the end of the day I was diagnosed with two rare and unrelated neurological disorders. Given what many people face, I was very lucky. I couldn't do everything, but I discovered that I could experience fitness in a new way. Even with my challenges, I could still feel good and get my body to perform better than it would if I didn't exercise. I am a lot healthier, due in no small part to doing regular workouts.

I still am vulnerable to tripping and falling, but I am OK. I reframed my training into what I can accomplish, not what I am unable to do. Fitness is a lifeline for me—and I have not allowed my health issues to interfere with a good quality of life. Exercise helps me feel better, function better, and enjoy my life. For that, I will be forever thankful.

CHAPTER SEVEN

GOOD
JOB!

WHAT COULD I possibly have to say on the topic of happiness and jobs? After all, except for a few summer jobs when I was growing up, I've always worked for myself. I'm an entrepreneur, not a management expert or HR professional.

That said, I have hired, or been involved in hiring, thousands of people—from personal trainers to front desk motivators to club construction personnel to leadership team members—to work at GoodLife Fitness. And I've always wanted every job to be engaging and, in turn, to engage the members we serve.

From the very first days of starting this company from scratch, I've always viewed service to community as going hand-in-hand with service and caring about our members. I've always looked for people who demonstrate an interest in their personal fitness and have a keen interest in helping other people get fit—and if they volunteer in the community, even better. Every single team member is an important part of our culture of helping people get healthy and stay healthy. We look to hire people who want to make a difference to the health and happiness of our country, people who care.

This is why I wince when I hear the statistics that nearly 70 percent of people are not happy in the work they're doing, or feel that they're not in the right job for their talents and interests. There's no question that today's workplaces need a massive happiness and job satisfaction overhaul. Since we spend so much of our life in our jobs—every weekday or more, decade after decade—this is an extremely important issue.

A QUESTION
OF CULTURE

I MENTIONED THE culture of engagement we strive for at GoodLife, and, to me, a positive workplace culture is paramount. People today want companies not only to deliver great services or products but also to be good corporate citizens. Studies show that people are more likely to do business with a company that gives liberally to philanthropic causes and gets involved in the community. People want to work for those kinds of companies.

What's often missed is that each of us also has a personal culture. Ask yourself, "What do I stand for? Who am I in relation to my family, my friends, my colleagues, and my community?" When you're considering working for a company, it's important to figure out if your personal values align with the company's values. If they don't, then that is the wrong company for you. If they do, jump in.

If you're an entrepreneur who wants to start your own company, or if you're already doing that, your personal culture comes into play there as well. As an entrepreneur, you need to have a passion for your business, and that passion is fed by creating a company that reflects your values and what you find most meaningful in the world. It's not enough to start a company because you think it will fill a market niche or that it will rapidly become profitable.

Those things are important; however, they are not the heart of a business's success. I've established these core values in my business: caring, happiness, integrity, trust, personal fitness, passion, and peak attitude.

If you're a business owner, you're going to be spending day and night nurturing that company. So make sure it's something you love, something that emerges from your deepest personal values—and that you create a workplace culture based on those values.

THE
"PERFECT JOB"

THE PERFECT JOB is the one we would do for free, a job we would feel so good doing, it wouldn't feel like work at all. However, life is never perfect. As is the case with exercise, maybe "good enough is good enough" with respect to their job works for many people who define their life in other ways.

I'm not suggesting we should give up on our dream of the ideal job. We can experience happiness in our job if we find something to love about it—some other benefit that may not be immediately obvious. For example, a lumberjack might appreciate the way working outdoors contributes to his fitness—no pencil pushing behind a desk for him. A waiter might find meaning in contributing to other people's happiness, for example, by serving a wonderful meal to a family celebrating a birthday.

Almost every job helps to make a difference in some way. After all, work is what puts food on the table and hockey skates on the feet and fingers on the piano keys and nest eggs in the nest. Figure out what that difference is and then be aware of it every time you go to work.

If you feel you're in the wrong job, it's still important to find something about it you enjoy, something that will keep you feeling positive—not because you want to put on a false front, but because, if you have positive energy, someone else will notice it. A reputation for giving your all will get you better reference letters. Finding something you like about the job you have, but don't really want, will help you in your quest for the job you do want.

TALENT AND ATTITUDE MAKE GOOD PARTNERS

TALENT IS A good thing—even a great thing. Perseverance and attitude make good partners. An ongoing openness to learning opens a world of opportunity throughout your lifetime.

Some people have a genetic predisposition for certain types of work, say, in music, sports, or math. Some people have strong personality traits that lead them to success at work. "People people" often excel in sales and PR—and make great fitness instructors!

Perhaps you want to start a business, or you want to advance in the company you're working for. Is there a genetic predisposition to be successful in business? I don't think so. To succeed in business requires learning a whole constellation of different skills. Some of the skills may come more easily than others (courtesy of the talent part), but success in almost any career usually comes down to that combination of perseverance and learning.

Aspiration is part of this. It's a really good quality to have, as well as clear goals and the drive to achieve them. When we aspire to something, however, our tendency is to pin our happiness on the achievement and neglect the happiness markers along the way. Instead of thinking, "When I achieve *x*, I'll be happy," why not find instances of happiness and satisfaction along the way to the goal? Feeling good about the steps you take toward achieving a goal increases the quality of your ultimate arrival—and where you go next. It's not the mountaintop alone that is inspiring; it's also the climb. Otherwise, people would just hire a helicopter to get to the top, and where's the thrill in that?

Studies show that the happiness you experience on the way to a goal is longer lasting than the happiness you feel when you actually achieve the goal. Why? Because when you achieve the goal, your mind turns to, "OK, what new goal can I aspire to now?" The intense happiness you feel at the point of achievement can be short-lived. However, it's also the case that the less intense moments of happiness that you experience on your way to a goal have been shown to accumulate in your body and your mind, and they result in a much more abiding sense of overall happiness.

Another thing about aspiration is that it can become a desire "to have it all." Our culture definitely tells us we can have it all. It's not true! How could we? We don't have the capacity to enjoy everything that could possibly happen to us. There are always going to be trade-offs. Anytime you say yes to something, you say no to something else. If you say yes to going to medical school, you're saying no to getting enough sleep or to long vacations. If you say yes to moving to a different city for a job opportunity, you're saying no to staying in the familiar.

WHAT DOES FITNESS
HAVE TO DO WITH WORK?

PHYSICAL FITNESS IS of paramount importance to you in your work and career. How so? In so many ways. Exercising regularly, whether at home or by getting out and participating in fitness activities with others, gives you a sense of control over your health and raises your self-esteem. A fit person walking into a job interview is a whole other creature than one slouching in and out of breath. If people make decisions about you in the first microseconds of an experience, the first impression you give a prospective employer could make all the difference.

In an interview I heard with the astronaut Chris Hadfield, he talked about the toll that being in space took on his body, and the fact that he had to be as fit as possible to even be considered to go into orbit. He indicated that being in space is stressful and not as glamorous as everyone thinks. He also said that it was entirely worth it. "Look what I got to do! See the earth from outer space and have an experience I will always remember."

Every job requires heroic efforts from time to time and staying power at the same time for daily routines. Having good physical stamina is key to surviving and thriving in such situations.

Consider what many corporations are actively doing to encourage employees to take exercise breaks on the job during lunch hours or after work. Employees appreciate this type of consideration for their wellness and look favourably on companies that offer their support. The benefit to the company is well documented. A fit workforce means fewer sick days, greater energy, and greater earnings.

THE BEST
YOU CAN BE

ANOTHER ATTITUDE I find useful in achieving work-related goals is striving not for perfection but to be the best you can be. It's the same with fitness, as I've mentioned earlier in the book. Don't strive for a non-existent perfection. Instead decide to be the best you can be. Doing your best will give you a deep sense of satisfaction.

Like aspiring to a goal, doing your best is often accomplished in small steps. If you're looking only for the really large milestones, you're not going to notice all the really neat things happening to you along the way. Having job-related or life-related goals will push you out of your comfort zone. That means you're going to have to trust yourself, and very often that involves taking small steps.

If, for example, you've just joined a fitness club after being out of shape for a long time, perhaps all you can do is five minutes on a treadmill or stationary bike. You may think that's a small step, but look how huge it really is. You have gone from being sedentary to putting your body into action.

Five minutes today becomes 10 minutes next week, and the 10 becomes 20, and one day you notice that you don't get out of breath anymore when you're doing chores like carrying grocery bags from your car to the kitchen or walking up some steps. That's when you realize that the small step you took to get in the door of that club was one of the biggest steps of your life.

It's like that with your life's work, too. The path to a job or career you enjoy is a series of small steps, and often the very first step is the one you will always remember because it's the step that put you on your path.

CHAPTER EIGHT

GOOD BODY, GOOD MIND

WE ALL KNOW we'll be healthier if we eat nutritious food, and we know our body will function better if we exercise. We should know, too, that fitness has as much impact on our brainpower as it does on bodies. Exercise creates a more efficient flow of oxygen to all parts of the body—and the brain is part of the body. Improved oxygen flow to the brain improves its capability for thinking.

Studies have shown that people who exercise regularly produce more work and score better in tests. They have a more optimistic outlook. They recover faster from anxiety and stress. A direct benefit of exercise is the ability to think more clearly, not only because of increased oxygen to the brain but also because a body that functions well allows the brain to focus on what it does best.

The body's way of coping with stress is through physical movement. If you're not moving, then you have to rely on the passage of time to take the stress away. As we know, in a society where stress is more common than the common cold, there's no time for recovery! If you're under stress, you're simply not as efficient. If you reduce the effects of stress with exercise, your brain is able to deal with the tasks at hand clearly and concisely.

Another way that exercise contributes to brainpower is by improving the quality of your sleep. When you're getting adequate exercise, you enter REM (rapid eye movement) sleep more quickly and have a deeper, more restful sleep overall. Your body is better able to repair itself naturally during sleep, not having to battle the tiredness that comes from chronic stress. Your body will do the real work of self-renewal. If you sleep better, you think better the next day.

CONTROL
YOUR MIND

WHEN YOU'RE RUNNING around frantically with too many deadlines, flustered, exasperated, and stressed out, you're not able to think as clearly as when you're calm, relaxed, and in control. Your heart can operate at 10 or 25 fewer beats per minute if you're in shape than it can if you're inactive. When your heart is beating at a lower rate, you are more in control, and your thinking is clearer.

This mental clarity arising from regular fitness helps fit people be more productive, make more money, and lead happier lives. Fit people have the good life, in every sense of the word. People who exercise regularly seem to be more in control than people who don't, just as a dog that gets a walk every day is brighter and more content.

Part of being fit is being able to concentrate and be goal-oriented. In the workplace this often translates into business success. Numerous studies show that fit people make more money. I remember one study from when I was in university showing that people who made over $60,000 worked out for six hours a week on average. Because fit people have a lower stress level and higher productivity, they are likely to become more accomplished at what they do and thus make more money.

Enlightened businesses know that fit employees benefit the company. That's why some employers pay for fitness programs for their employees, and some even have fitness facilities on-site. This isn't just a perk. These companies know that any edge they can get in the competitive marketplace is worth it.

This is true not just of corporate workplaces. Let's take another example: airplanes. Why does a pilot have to be fitter than a bus driver? If anything, flying a plane is a less physical job than driving a bus. The pilot often just guides the airplane using automatic controls. So why do airlines insist that pilots stay fit? Because the pilots need to be able to control stress, stay cool under pressure, and think clearly. You might say that so does a bus driver, and that's true. However, pilots are in the sky. My point is that the higher the mental sophistication needed for a task, the more you need to be fit overall.

Let's take astronauts as an example. An astronaut gets strapped into a capsule and doesn't move more than two or three feet in one direction for days on end. Yet NASA makes sure that its astronauts are excellent physical specimens. Why? Going into space is stressful both physically and mentally, and in that high-risk environment you need your wits about you. John Glenn, 77 years old when he last went into space, had the fitness level of a 50-year-old man.

If you're fit, your body is in tune with your environment. You have higher self-esteem and self-awareness. If you feel in control of your body, you'll also feel in control of your mind. You'll tend to believe you can do things. A good basic level of fitness allows you to enjoy dancing or playing sports or walking on the beach. Good fun in fitness activities can lead to good thinking.

EXERCISE
AFFECTS LEARNING

IT'S WELL KNOWN that active children get higher marks in school. That's why I support and applaud the fact that schools are encouraging children to be active and are making sure that they get time in the gym and outdoors as part of their school day. There is nothing like a great game of tag and filling up the lungs with fresh air to make kids feel more alert and energized.

Our brainpower resides in our body! Sometimes we forget that the brain is a physical organ. So, to me, mind/body unity is a given fact. Children who exercise during the school day will be happier, readier to learn, and healthier overall.

I developed the GoodLife Kids Foundation to support innovative fitness programs aimed at children. We provide educational resources and funding to interesting programs, many of which happen in remoter areas of the country. Another thing I committed my company to is offering free membership in the clubs to teenagers during the summer. To date, more than 100,000 enthusiastic teens have spent their summers working out (in addition to their summer jobs and leisure time). For a fitter and healthier generation to come up behind today's current adults, we need to attend to the exercise needs of the young. We need to leave what I call "a fitness legacy."

There's a key point for you to remember, whether you're a parent wanting to encourage your kids to spend time outside or a teacher looking for ways to incorporate physical movement during the school day: it's not hard to get kids to kick a ball around, or to get them to run around the block, or to have them do some stretching in the classroom. Kids don't care whether the exercise is elaborate or not—they just want to have fun. A turning point for me in terms of fitness came in my last year of high school. We went running every day for eight weeks. I remember being the slowest runner at the beginning and in the top five by the end of the eight weeks. I remember how much better I felt every day. I didn't set out to get into the top five. I actually hated having to run. I thought I was just a big, slow guy. I did play hockey and high school football, but running at that time was not a big thing for me. As I said earlier, my father died when I was a child, so, coming from a single-parent household, I had to work at part-time jobs. When I was in high school, I worked 25 to 30 hours a week. I will never forget the slow, incremental improvements I made as a runner and how good I felt as my body became more energetic and efficient—different from the sports I played because it was always available, free, and fun.

Teachers have an opportunity to be role models to their students, supporting a culture that includes exercise in their daily lives. We all know of the studies that say sitting at a desk for more than three hours at a time for adults in the workforce leads to an increased risk of diabetes, heart disease, and weight gain. Do we expect it is any less dangerous for our children just to sit around? On average, Canadian children spend two-thirds of their daytime hours being sedentary. Scientific data aside, common sense tells us this is not healthy. Kids need to move. Marks go up just like adult incomes do when kids get some time for fitness breaks and exercise in school.

Fitness programs for children, in comparison with a lot of other things in our society, don't have to take a lot of time or cost a lot of money. Fitness should be public policy. Good bodies lead to good brains. If we're going to meet the challenges of the 21st century, we need as many good brains as we can get!

IN-THE-BODY
MINDFULNESS

I HAVE OFTEN thought of certain kinds of exercise as akin to what can happen in meditation. Yoga and Tai Chi definitely promote a meditational mindset. However, even just going for a walk and letting your mind float can be a meditative experience, as can allowing your mind to empty itself of thoughts and concerns as you walk on a treadmill or StairMaster or work on a rowing machine, following your breath as you do so. We are in an alpha brainwave state when our conscious mind quiets down and we let random thoughts just flow through in a relaxed way. This is the brainwave pattern we feel when we're daydreaming or floating in a swimming pool. Alpha brainwaves trigger the relaxation response.

Do you see what this means? If you can get your mind into an alpha pattern while exercising, your body will benefit from the physical exercise itself, and your relaxed mind will release more of those feel-good endorphins.

Some meditative techniques ask people to disassociate from the body, or to feel they are floating above their body. Perhaps these techniques can be useful in a spiritual sense. However, I prefer to think that mindfulness puts us fully into our bodies, which is why I prefer techniques and suggestions that allow us to sink into our bodies and really feel them. The body is the house where we live: our brainpower, our emotions, our thoughts, and our spirit. Caring for the whole you starts with the body.

I like the idea that regular exercise is a way of honouring our entire being. It's a way of saying yes to ourselves. It's a way of allowing us to actually show up in our lives, to be present to our loved ones. When you partner with your own body, you are partnering with all the other parts of you as well. There is no split between mind and body—there is just you!

ONE OF OUR CLUB MEMBERS ON PHYSICAL AND MENTAL FITNESS

DR. LORI T.

FITNESS NOT ONLY has improved my own life but also has enhanced my ability to save lives as an emergency physician. And it has made me a more effective university professor. Through personal training I have gained the skills to develop and maintain excellent upper body strength. Having a strong left arm is critically important during intubation (inserting an artificial breathing tube). This strength, combined with technique, allowed me to save a man's life when I performed an extremely difficult intubation. Strength and fitness have increased my success at numerous other emergency procedures as well. I often encourage the resident physicians whom I teach to pursue fitness and build strength to become more adept in their field.

As a physician in a major trauma centre, I "speed walk" up to 12 kilometres per shift, attending to a multitude of patients as well as supervising residents and medical students. It is imperative that I maintain top cardiovascular and muscle conditioning to keep up this grueling pace. Fitness has helped me acquire endurance and the high level of energy required to meet the physical and mental demands of emergency work— especially shift work.

My additional role as an assistant professor makes it essential that I not only keep informed of new developments in medicine but also continually review the basics to enable me to instruct many students and residents every day. I have developed a way to study during exercise. Twenty to 30 minutes on the treadmill has become useful time for reviewing and refreshing my storehouse of medical knowledge. I have become a curiosity at my fitness club, memorizing and reviewing over a thousand study cards I designed for use during exercise. I even used this study system to help me attain my board certification in emergency medicine.

CHAPTER NINE

GOOD ENOUGH
IS GOOD ENOUGH

EXPECTATIONS CAN BE tricky. On the one hand, we're told by many personal development experts that putting too many expectations on ourselves isn't healthy. On the other hand, we're told by other personal development experts that, if we set goals for ourselves, we also have to work to reach those goals.

I want to chart a middle course between these two contrasting viewpoints. There are ways to have good expectations of yourself without imposing too many on yourself. The key to this, I think, is that we learn both to dream and be realistic. I think the path to happiness is in the balance of dreams with reality. So the first point I want us to consider here is: What is a good expectation to have?

In my years since 1979 as a fitness club owner, I have developed a phrase I use with my staff and with the club members—*Good enough is good enough*. To me, this is the very essence of a fit and healthy lifestyle—to know when you've reached the point of being "good enough" in terms of your health and well-being.

The average age of our members at GoodLife in the year

2014 is 34. The people who join our clubs range all the way from teenagers to people in their 60s, 70s, and even 80s. The baby-boomer generation makes up a big portion of membership in fitness clubs, too. If any member were to go to any magazine rack and thumb through the pages of a fitness or lifestyle magazine, they would find articles telling them how to be perfect. Articles on how to have the best abdominals or the best biceps, how to run a marathon or do a triathlon at any age. The magazines go on and on about perfection. They give examples of people who have done incredible things. They create a huge guilt syndrome, as if people who don't already feel bad enough that they weren't good at sports in high school and never made any of the teams aren't also going to feel inadequate every time they pick up one of these magazines and see these "perfect" bodies. They're always faced with the fact that the model in the photos is 20 years younger than they are, or 20 pounds lighter, or just perceived better.

I try to instill in my staff the importance of telling people there is a level of fitness that is good enough. "Good enough" means that your expectations for your health and fitness can be both good and realistic. "Good enough" is the level of fitness you need to have a healthy and rewarding life. To use an analogy, there's a maximum speed limit on highways because if you drive a lot faster than that, you risk getting seriously injured or even killed, and there's a minimum speed limit because if you drive more slowly than that, you'll also be at risk of an accident because someone may ram into you. In terms of fitness, one extreme is to think you need to work out six hours a day, and you push and push, because you want that body you saw in a magazine. An athlete always verges on injury in order to be exceptional. It's so competitive in high-level sport that athletes always have to push their limits, and so they risk both injury and mental burnout. The other extreme is not being active. Sooner or later you're going to get injured, or you'll have more illnesses, or people will pass you by because they're more successful and enjoy things more.

As an average person, you don't need to worry about getting even close to the speed limit. In our clubs we frequently get people asking us, "What if I burn out with exercise?" If you're the type of person who's going to burn out with exercise, it will be from trying to do too much for too long. For most of us, this is not an issue. You're much more likely not to do enough. However, you really only need to do strength exercises two or three times a week, or cardiovascular exercises two or three times a week, or a combination. You might do fitness classes that work the whole body. For example, using the Fit Fix formula we employ at GoodLife, you would warm up on cardio for five to ten minutes, and then you would do one set of weight/strength exercises per body part to success over 8 to 12 repetitions—6 to 12 exercises in total. Just 20 to 30 minutes in total for strength and cardio training three times a week—that's all you need to do. It seems almost too simple, but it works.

What we try to do with new people in our clubs is find out their needs and goals and when they would like to achieve those goals. Then we establish sensible parameters to help them get there so they can develop some good expectations for themselves. The key thing is to make the parameters realistic, so the person can feel it's worthwhile to do the exercises. We break everything down into reasonable goals. When the person reaches the goals, we say, "That's good. Now all you have to do is keep doing that for the rest of your life. Maintaining where you are is a lot easier than getting there." That's why I say, "Good enough is good enough."

THREE STAGES
TO BECOMING FIT

THERE ARE THREE stages in becoming fit.

The first stage is to stop getting worse. As soon as you stop getting worse, applaud yourself. If you stop putting on weight, that's a victory, even though you may still be overweight. If you stop yourself from losing any further muscle mass and strength, that's a victory. Most people never recognize that. Stage one of "good enough is good enough" could be that you're 40 pounds overweight and you stop gaining more—that's fantastic!

The second stage is to begin reversing the damage. You decide how much you want to reverse. Say you are 40 pounds overweight and you decide to take off 20 pounds. When you get to that point, celebrate the victory. Then all you have to do is maintain that level. If you're doing the same weights two or three times a week, you reach your goal, and you keep doing the same thing from year to year, in fitness terms it means you're not getting any older. If you've taken your 20 pounds off and have increased your strength by 100 percent, which almost everyone can do in six weeks, you have reduced your age in terms of your actual fitness age. Chronological age is one thing; actual age is another. If you can do the same things at 40 that you could do at 30—fitness-wise, you are 30.

The third stage is simply maintenance. That's what I mean by "good enough is good enough." A small number of the general population, probably under 2 percent, want to go to their maximum fitness levels. However, to be fit you don't have to be at your maximum fitness level.

Many people quit fitness programs because they don't realize that just stopping getting worse is a good thing. Or they lay expectations on themselves that are too aggressive and too fast and aren't satisfied when they don't achieve them. Or they keep setting further and further goals, when instead they should be saying, "I'm OK."

If you fit within the body-fat and strength parameters for your body type, if you can do what you want to do in life, if your stress level is controlled by the fitness activities you do, that is good enough. It should be a non-issue in your life. So when you get to 20 percent body fat, you don't have to push to get to 10 percent. You might just say, "I'm happy with 20 percent because I'm healthy, I look good, and I feel good." You don't have to become the next perfect bikini figure or the next Mr. Hercules. You have to be who you are. You are a 10 already!

STAYING
MOTIVATED

PEOPLE OFTEN ASK me about motivation. The best way I know to stay motivated in fitness is to chase "good enough" instead of chasing perfection. You realize that you don't have to be perfect. To use another driving analogy, how many people can drive like a professional auto racer? Not very many. So does that mean you shouldn't drive at all? Of course not!

A lot of people would like to be millionaires, but how many are willing to pay the price in terms of the hours and effort needed to actually become one? That's why it's so attractive to dream about winning a lottery or answering the million-dollar question on *Who Wants to Be a Millionaire?* Well, you can't win a lottery that helps your body, but you can win the health and happiness game with "good enough is good enough."

Another big component in motivating yourself is to be happy that you're not deteriorating and becoming decrepit— or, even more importantly, to realize that you can turn back the calendar on your age. Imagining the months going backward on a calendar can be a powerful motivator. Most people can get to that stage within three to six months. If you make your "real" age 30 in terms of fitness, and you can stay 30 until you're 55, isn't that exciting to contemplate? Every year, the day before my birthday, I weigh myself to make sure I'm the same as I was a year ago. On the day of my birthday I give myself my annual physical check-up. I test myself on the cardiovascular equipment to check that I've maintained my fitness levels, and I do the same with our strength circuit. Sometimes I even do better than the year before.

A training routine for good health and fitness should always be done in cycles. Think of it as waves on a beach, coming one after another. Here is the type of cycle I use:

SEPTEMBER–NOVEMBER
My strongest focus is on strength training. At the same time I maintain my cardiovascular fitness level as good enough.

DECEMBER–MARCH
During the winter months I tend to be in a holding pattern. I love to swim, so I do it as much as I can. I keep my strength and my cardiovascular fitness at roughly the same level. This is great psychologically because it means I don't always feel I have to improve. I can go through phases where I maintain one thing and focus on another rather than trying to do everything at once.

APRIL–AUGUST

This is when I make my cardio workouts harder. This makes the summer an excellent time for me to concentrate on cardio while still maintaining my strength.

The idea behind training cycles is to focus primarily on one part of your training at a time while maintaining the others. You'll become stronger, fitter, and faster if you train in cycles. Your body needs periods of recovery and rest. These periods allow you to focus more intensely when you work harder on the other areas. Training cycles allow you to adapt your fitness routines to your body's needs, your favourite sports, and your particular lifestyle.

Most people's resting heart rate goes up about one beat per year. So if mine doesn't go up, I'm not getting older. If it goes up only one beat in five years, I'm still staying younger. Let's say you're 50 and your resting heart rate is 65. If the average is 78, that's good. If you exercise and, six months later, your resting heart rate is down to 60, you've just shaved five years off your fitness age. You're not 50 anymore, you're 45 or younger. Resting heart rates can vary, but the improvement is what counts.

Once you have gone through the learning curve of becoming fit—learning how to strength-train, become flexible, and do cardiovascular training—you can just keep doing the same thing. You won't see articles in magazines that say, "Don't change. What you're doing is fine." People may think this could be boring, to keep doing the same thing at the good enough level. Well, so is brushing your teeth, but it's nice to have good teeth. So is washing, but it's nice to smell good and look good. The point is that such a fitness routine is non-stressful and easily maintained. A major benefit is that you give it a small amount of time and reap a huge payback.

Magazine publishers can't sell magazines to you if you think you're OK. Sure, we will always encounter problems in life, and it's not necessarily a bad thing to look for advice in magazines or books. (Like mine, for example!) My point is that you should be wary of those magazines, TV shows, books, and movies that flaunt perfection, because perfection does not exist. Good enough is good enough says, "I'm OK." The body is wonderful. It doesn't need perfection. It just needs a level where it can work well and you can feel good. It's also OK to ask for help. I use a personal trainer myself whenever I can. Personal trainers are a fantastic way to stay on course. Everyone can benefit from another opinion and the extra motivation.

GOOD ENOUGH
IS BALANCE

BY MAKING A decision to be fit and then recognizing that good enough is good enough, you can balance everything that is important in your life. You can achieve this balance because you have a high level of self-esteem as a result of taking control of yourself and having some good expectations about reaching a good level of well-being. Regardless of what anyone else says on the subject, it is widely agreed that part of balance is the ability to cope and deal with things in a positive manner. Fitness allows you to cope with anything that comes your way.

When you achieve balance, you establish healthier priorities in your life. When you become fit and your body gets in sync with you, you find that balance begins to extend into other areas of your life. You're not consumed by your work life. You find time for family and friends, for recreation, solitude, and reflection. In so many cases I have seen people's decision to pursue fitness carry over into every other aspect of their lives. It's not important whether you do your fitness routines in the morning, the afternoon, or the evening. Do them when it suits you to do them. When you know what times you are going to devote to your fitness, it will help you establish a time frame for everything else. Make your workout appointments with yourself—this is a most important commitment. If you decide to work out before breakfast, then you know what time you're going to get up. If you decide to work out in the evening, you know what time you need to leave the office or what time dinner will be. Fitness routines will help you establish healthy patterns.

Why do I think fitness should be such a priority in your life? Because your life is a priority. When you decide to be fit, you've decided to take self-control. And self-control leads to balance. When you listen to your body, you also listen to your head, your heart, and your spirit. When you achieve a state of balance, you become aware that there is no split. You are one whole organism. Everything you do to achieve health and fitness has an effect on your mind, your emotions, and your inner peace.

When you are under stress, as most of us are in this society, with its technological advances and rapid pace of change, your body and spirit deserve the recovery that exercise brings. You deserve to burn off any negativity and anxiety and the effects of overwork and other life challenges. Fitness will help you get through tough times. When life throws you a curveball, if you're healthy and fit you'll find it easier to maintain your equilibrium.

It begins with the body. Think of yourself as a house. Your fit body is your foundation. An unfit body is an unstable foundation. If your intellect and emotions are the walls, and your foundation is fit, those walls stay up straight and help you hold your treasures inside. If the walls are vulnerable because your foundation is shaky, the house could fall apart. Think of your soul as the roof. To be truly self-actualized, everything below the roof needs to be in good working order. Everything works together to make the dwelling place that is you.

Something interesting happens when you think in terms of having good expectations rather than having unwieldy ones. By keeping your focus on what is both good and realistic in your life, you can actually find yourself on the path to having the kind of life where there is so much good around you and in you that you can knock it out of the park! That's happiness!

CONNECTEDNESS

IT'S ALMOST A cliché these days—so many are saying, "Everything is connected. We are all connected to each other." However, science is increasingly suggesting that this is true.

A few years ago, I had the honour of introducing Deepak Chopra at a speaking event. Deepak comes from a long history of medicine in India known as Ayurveda, which has all kinds of ideas about metabolism, diet, balance, movement, serenity, and meditation. At one point, Deepak and I got talking about the idea of the physical universe being connected to everything that exists. He commented that anytime you're talking to someone, you're sharing 75 atoms. They have within themselves 75 "pieces" of you at the atomic level, and you have 75 "pieces" of them, just from the air you breathe.

I'm not sure exactly where Deepak got this information, or whether his Ayurvedic understanding of "atom" is the same as in the Western world, or how he arrived at the number 75. However, he was certainly right about the fact that, when you and I are in a room together, we are sharing the same air. OK, you may protest at this point that breathing the same air means we could all catch a cold that's going around, but that actually makes my point. The reason many people in a room might catch a cold is precisely that we're connected by the air we breathe. On a more serious note, we realize that we are all connected through our common humanity. We are also connected to the animal kingdom and to the history of everything that has happened before we were even born.

We know that we humans share 99 percent of the same DNA as chimpanzees and that compatible DNA between ourselves and almost all creatures can be found to some degree. If you went on an archaeological dig, you would realize that you were standing on the same ground where people stood thousands of years ago. If you went camping and drank from a stream, it could be a stream that existed when the first hunter-gatherers stopped to refresh themselves. Ancient cultures connect to modern cultures; mountains have been around for millennia; hundreds of millions of people over hundreds of thousands of years have seen the sun rise and the moon rise. We have looked at the same stars. We have told many of the same stories. We pass ourselves on in the DNA of our children. So, to me, the sense of connection is much wider than just realizing that we should be out there "making connections" with people in a social sense. There is a far deeper sense of connection, and nature is so great at giving us these feelings that ground us, that make us feel part of something much larger than ourselves.

I call this "living life with a wide lens." This connected approach can lead to the feeling of being at home wherever you are, being at home in your own body and having your place here. Wise people throughout history have described this feeling of connection as a form of happiness. If in fact we are all connected with our thoughts and genes, we can continue to build a happiness connection in the world.

APPRECIATION

ANOTHER HAPPINESS QUALITY linked to the idea of connection I've just talked about is a sense of appreciation. Do we do enough in our lives to give ourselves a sense of appreciation toward ourselves? To know that our life matters just because we exist? Do we do enough to appreciate the presence of others in our lives? To appreciate other creatures?

I remember almost getting knocked over by a kangaroo that hopped up right behind me while I was running in Australia at night. Its tail went thump, thump, thump, and then it hopped right past me. I could feel the wind as it passed. I was afraid at first of possibly falling or being run over by this big red 'roo, but I sure did appreciate the beauty of this creature with its incredible bounce. To Aussies, seeing a kangaroo is commonplace. To me it was a moment of wonder and appreciation. If you learn to expect that each day you will see some good things to appreciate, you will see them.

CREATIVITY

CREATIVITY IS ANOTHER way to knock it out of the park. Most people think creativity is only for artists or musicians or computer geniuses. Yes, those individuals are definitely creative. So are you! Every person has a unique life story; everyone has something he or she is good at; every one of us can come up with a different way to do things, whether it's trying a new recipe, walking home by a different route, or going on vacation somewhere we have never been before. Creativity is about doing new and different things. It doesn't have to be a painting or the starring role on Broadway. It can just be a little game we play with ourselves each day when we ask, "What could I do today that is different from yesterday? Is there a better, more interesting way?"

Most people think creativity is tied to talent. That's certainly true of some forms of creativity. It is unlikely that I will ever be able to paint the way the Group of Seven did, and you definitely do not want to hear me recite Shakespeare! Far more important than talent, however, is perseverance and attitude. That's certainly what's needed when you're starting or running a business or your life. There is research that shows that even with just modest talent, a person can reach a high level of competency. People are talking about the 10,000-hour factor. If a person spends that many hours doing something over an extended period of time, he or she will gain mastery of whatever the activity is. Maybe that sounds like a lot to you: 10,000 hours. Well, that's for mastery. The biggest gains, for example, in fitness are in the first 100 hours. Take a look at your job. If you've been there several years, you've likely reached the 10,000-hour mark. If you've been exercising for several years, and you make it part of your daily routine, you're likely approaching several hundred hours. If you've been raising children, by the time your children are teenagers you've done more than 10,000 hours of parenting. We don't give ourselves nearly enough credit for the things we do, the things we persist at over time, the parts of our lives that require us to be creative and flexible.

OPPORTUNITIES

ANOTHER WAY OF recognizing, and expecting, happiness in our lives is to be aware of opportunities when they present themselves. If you've always wanted to do something, and the opportunity arises to do it, then do it (provided it's not something criminal or something that would harm others). I remember getting my first bank loan for GoodLife when I was intent on opening my first club. Most of the banks turned me down flat. Finally, a banker named Brian Smith of TD Bank gave me the loan.

I told him, "You know that I'm not sure if my snowplowing business could pay this back just yet. It might take a long time."

He said, "I know that, but I've read your character and your determination, and I know that you will pay it back."

He provided me with the opportunity of getting that very first loan, which, in turn, provided an opportunity to open that very first club, enabling me eventually to give up the snowplowing business and focus on fitness. Years later, Brian saw an opportunity in me that would benefit him. He had me come as a "celebrity guest" to the Chamber of Commerce where he could "show me off" as a business success story he had supported. He would say to people, "I believed in the business because I believed in the guy. I bet on him as a person, and we won." He had good expectations of me.

I'm not telling you this in order to brag or to make myself seem special. It's just an illustration of the power of acting on an opportunity, and how it leads to happiness. Brian was happy to have played a role in the creation of GoodLife; I was happy to have met someone who believed in me and took a chance on me when everyone else said no. And later, as the clubs opened one by one, customers were made happy by the fact that they had somewhere to work out and to meet others who were also interested in working out.

I often reflect on how lucky I was to have Jack Fairs as a professor in my physical education studies. Jack taught me about the relationship between mind and body. His philosophy about how the body affects the mind and vice versa has been a philosophical undercurrent in my business and has shaped so many of the programs created at the clubs. Back in my university days, Jack was a professor who offered me the opportunity to learn, and I saw that he had something very special to offer. Rather than slacking off or skipping classes, as some university students are tempted to do, I decided to absorb everything I could from this man.

Even some of the toughest things in my life have been disguised opportunities.

Losing my father at such a young age gave me the opportunity to learn resilience and survival skills in a tough economic situation. I'm not saying that my father's death was a good thing; it certainly wasn't—I would have preferred to grow up with my father in my life. What I'm saying is that his death created an opportunity to grow up and mature faster and to learn some very important life skills, such as getting a job after school hours—an unwanted opportunity, but nevertheless one that helped create the kind of person I am today.

Having an autistic daughter has also created unusual opportunities for me—the opportunity to learn alternate ways of communicating with her, to learn about compassion and patience, to learn about loving her exactly as she is. I discovered qualities in myself that I never knew were there. Patience was never my strength as a young man, but Kilee taught me about patience. She also taught me about joy as I saw each and every step she made in progressing to the best of her abilities.

Another great opportunity has been the chance to support the leading-edge research of Dr. Derrick MacFabe on autism and to see the research team achieving results that are being shared around the world. I have had the opportunity to meet other parents of autistic children. I have had the opportunity to speak publicly about autism. I have had the opportunity to share the message that this condition is far from hopeless, and even though Kilee still has her setbacks and I have my challenges in parenting her, her presence in my life has been an opportunity that has brought a deep sense of meaning, even beyond my passion for fitness. A deep sense of meaning is perhaps the most lasting kind of happiness of all.

CELEBRATION

LASTLY, IN THIS chapter, I want to talk about celebration. Isn't life a lot happier when you have something to celebrate? Don't just think of birthdays or anniversaries or births or graduations as times to celebrate. Imagine if you saw celebration as something you did really often: celebrating losing two pounds, celebrating going to a dance when all along you thought you were not that great a dancer, celebrating being able to take a vacation, celebrating after doing a challenging hike or a charity run, celebrating a friend's promotion at work. My good friend Tony de Leede says that every day is a holiday, and every meal is a feast. Celebrate life itself!

An attitude of celebration, the idea that every day can bring something to celebrate, will help you develop what I call the happiness habit. You don't have to go buy a cake or a card every time you encounter one of these celebratory moments, just a quiet acknowledgement that brings a smile to your face will do. Give yourself the good expectation that celebration can make your life a lot happier. Sometimes, do make the celebration big—if you've set a goal to improve your muscle strength and you find you have so much more energy, celebrate! Go out dancing with that new energy! Do your happy dance!

Recently, I was lucky enough to find a brilliant surgeon

who totally rebuilt my wild toes. I had him straighten the bones in my toes, not out of vanity—more for the idea of being able to function better on my feet and have 90 percent less pain. I don't know what the long term will bring or whether the arthritis will again establish itself in my feet, but at this moment I'm celebrating this improvement to my quality of life right now. It's helping me to dance and ski better, too. I have "happy feet!"

In fact, I think happiness is a dance, or is like one of life's key elements: water. Just as there are many forms of water, including snow, so there are many versions of happiness. It's not something linear that just shows up and stays there without changing. It is fluid; it has rhythm and flow. Sometimes it hides, but it never disappears entirely. It is there waiting to be discovered right now in the life you are living at this very moment. Expect it. You'll find it. Happiness is a dance—I like that!

ONE OF OUR CLUB MEMBERS ON GOOD EXPECTATIONS

MILES K.

MY LIFE HAS changed for the better since getting involved with fitness. I have found that it takes courage to make big changes in life. Starting a fitness program was not an easy task for me. Most people know they should probably join a fitness club but are often too intimidated to take the first step. I used to think that I had to lose weight on my own before I could even be seen by other people in a gym. But when I joined the gym, I realized that everyone else there was just trying to do the same thing. It was a question of taking control of my life. It has made such a huge difference in my personal and professional life. I'm better able to set targets and work toward accomplishing larger goals, both personally and in my job. Let's face it: Life is about getting a little further ahead.

You just need the right motivational tools and the stamina to get there. I really am living the good life!

To be your best,
To be what you could be,
All you have to do is be.
You have to be as strong as you can be.
You need a heart that pumps and is not blocked,
Lungs that inhale and exhale with deep, full breaths,
Legs that stride and run,
Arms that pump,
A straight back,
Good skin, shining eyes.
Make your body your foundation,
The foundation of the good life.
Be your best,
But keep in mind—
Always—
Good enough is good enough.

—PATCH

125 GOOD REASONS TO EXERCISE

EXERCISE MAKES SENSE, BECAUSE IT

1. increases your self-confidence and your self-esteem
2. improves your digestion
3. helps you sleep better
4. gives you more energy
5. adds a healthy glow to your complexion
6. strengthens your immune system
7. improves your body shape
8. burns up extra calories
9. tones and firms your muscles
10. provides more muscle definition
11. improves circulation and helps lower blood pressure
12. lifts your spirits
13. reduces tension and stress
14. helps you to lose weight and keeps you at your right body weight
15. makes you limber/flexible

16. builds strength
17. improves endurance
18. increases lean muscle tissue in your body
19. improves your appetite for healthy food
20. alleviates menstrual cramps
21. alters and improves muscle chemistry
22. increases your metabolic rate
23. improves coordination and balance
24. improves your posture
25. eases and may eliminate back problems and pain
26. alters the way your body uses calories
27. lowers your resting heart rate
28. increases muscle size by increasing muscle fibres
29. improves storage of glycogen
30. enables your body to use nutrients more efficiently
31. increases the enzymes in the body that burn fat
32. increases the number and size of mitochondria in each muscle cell
33. strengthens your bones
34. increases the concentration of myoglobin, which carries oxygen, in the skeletal muscles
35. enhances oxygen transport throughout the body
36. improves liver function
37. increases the speed of muscle contraction and therefore reaction time
38. enhances feedback through the nervous system
39. strengthens the heart

40. improves blood flow through the body
41. helps alleviate varicose veins
42. increases maximum cardiac output because of an increase in stroke volume
43. increases contractility of the heart's ventricles
44. increases the weight of the heart
45. increases heart size
46. improves contractile function of the whole heart
47. makes calcium transport in the heart and the entire body more efficient
48. helps prevent heart disease
49. increases the level of HDL (high-density lipoprotein)
50. decreases LDL (low-density lipoprotein)
51. decreases cholesterol
52. decreases triglycerides
53. increases total hemoglobin, which carries oxygen in the red blood cells
54. increases the blood's alkaline reserve (buffering capacity)
55. improves the body's ability to remove lactic acid
56. improves the body's ability to decrease heart rate after exercise
57. increases the number of capillaries that are open during exercise as opposed to when at rest
58. improves blood flow to the active muscles at the peak of training

59. enhances the function of the cardiovascular system
60. enhances the function of the cardio-respiratory system
61. improves efficiency in breathing
62. increases respiratory capacity
63. improves ventilation of the alveoli (air sacs in the lungs) for greater oxygen consumption
64. lessens sensitivity to the buildup of CO_2 (carbon dioxide)
65. improves breathing, in that less ventilation is required per litre of O_2 (oxygen) consumption
66. improves bone metabolism
67. decreases the chances of developing osteoporosis
68. improves the development and strength of connective tissue
69. lowers your risk of death from cancer
70. improves resistance to infectious diseases
71. enhances neuromuscular relaxation
72. enables you to relax more quickly and completely
73. alleviates depression
74. improves emotional stability
75. enhances clarity of the mind
76. makes you feel good
77. increases the efficiency of your sweat glands
78. enables you to stay warmer in colder environments
79. helps you respond more effectively to heat, since sweating begins at a lower body temperature
80. improves your body's overall composition

81. increases body density

82. decreases fat tissue more easily

83. helps you make your body more agile

84. increases your positive attitude about yourself and your life

85. increases the level of the hormone norepinephrine, which boosts the spirits

86. stimulates release of hormones that alleviate pain

87. alleviates constipation

88. increases the efficiency with which adrenaline is used, resulting in more energy

89. enables you to meet new friends and develop fulfilling relationships

90. enables you to socialize at the same time that you are getting into shape

91. helps you move past self-imposed limitations

92. gives you a greater appreciation for life because you feel better about yourself

93. enables you to enjoy all types of physical activities more

94. makes your clothes look better on you

95. makes it easier to exercise consistently because you like the way you look and feel and don't want to lose it

96. gives you a greater desire to participate 100 percent in life—to take more risks—as a result of increased confidence and self-esteem

97. improves athletic performance

98. enhances sexual performance

99. improves the whole quality of your life

100. helps you live longer and better, giving you an extra hour of life for every hour of exercise

101. is the greatest tune-up for the body

102. reduces joint discomfort

103. increases your range of motion

104. gives you a feeling of control or mastery over your life and the belief that you can create any reality that you want

105. stimulates and improves concentration

106. brings colour to your cheeks

107. decreases appetite when you work out for 20 minutes to one hour

108. gets your mind off irritations

109. stimulates a feeling of well-being and accomplishment

110. invigorates the body and mind

111. is a wonderful way to enjoy nature and the great outdoors

112. increases the body's awareness of itself

113. reduces or prevents boredom

114. increases your awareness of your gait

115. enables you to move from left-brain to right-brain thinking

116. can change the electrical activity in the brain from beta to alpha waves

117. increases your ability to solve problems more easily, and often effortlessly

118. gives you a clearer perspective on ideas, issues, problems, and challenges

119. releases blockages and limitations in thinking

120. affords you the opportunity to experience your fullest potential

121. reduces illness

122. helps you live longer

123. makes you feel better each and every day

124. makes you feel more alive in your spirit

125. makes people look at you and say, "Wow! You look great!"

ACKNOWLEDGEMENTS

I would like to recognize the long-time dedication of my professional advisers Henry Berg, Bill Shanks, and Andy MacLaren, who have supported me since the early days.

I could not have made this journey into the demanding world of book publishing without the help and support of many individuals. My thanks to:

Sharon Lindenburger, who functioned as my trusted "scribe," helping me find the right words. Megan Cameron, who kept this book project on track, kept me motivated to get it done, and encouraged me throughout. And Donald G. Bastian, of Bastian Publishing Services, who believed in this project and guided the creation of the book with great care, sensitivity, and patience.

DAVID PATCHELL-EVANS

WELCOME TO GOODLIFE FITNESS

For the latest on Group Exercise programs, Health Centre services, Corporate Wellness, Personal Training, Member Rewards, JUMP! Child Minding, club locations, contests, and corporate information, visit our website at goodlifefitness.com

twitter.com/goodlifefitness

facebook.com/goodlifefitness

CONTENTS

GETTING STARTED

IT MAKES PERFECT sense to be healthy and fit!

First, let me offer my congratulations. You've made the important decision to make room in your life for this new priority so that you can look after yourself and enjoy a high quality of life in the future.

Now all that's needed is for you to establish your goals. When you write them down, they become real, so fill them in right here.

MY FITNESS GOALS FOR A
HEALTHIER, HAPPIER LIFE

WRITE DOWN YOUR top five goals that will make a difference in your life and the date by which you want to achieve them:

GOALS	MONTH, YEAR
1.	
2.	
3.	
4.	
5.	

Add any other goals that come to mind that you would like to achieve:

. . . .

. . . .

. . . .

. . . .

Lastly, it would be great to have someone witness your goals and timeline so that you have someone on your team to support you in your journey to good health.

Signed by your Supportive Witness!

_____

All the best,

Patch

ABOUT GOODLIFE
GoodLife's Vision

OUR VISION IS to give all Canadians the opportunity to live a fit and healthy good life. Our vision resonates with our passion to help more Canadians get off the couch and discover the benefits of a more active lifestyle. Experts are now describing sitting as "the new smoking," and the World Health Organization has now identified physical inactivity as the fourth cause of death on the planet. We want you to live longer. We want you to live healthier with a better quality of life.

How are we doing this?

- We have introduced more fitness club models to broaden the types of memberships available, such as our low-cost Fit4Less by GoodLife option.
- We are continually adding more locations to create greater convenience, such as Energie Cardio and Econofitness in Quebec.
- We offer free teen memberships during the summer months and a granting program through our GoodLife Kids Foundation to get young Canadians off to the right start.

WE ARE COMMITTED to great service and beautiful clubs to keep our members coming to their chosen club on a regular basis.

We want you to use your club as much as possible so you will succeed in reaching your fitness goals. That fulfills our vision.

GoodLife's Core Values
CARING | TRUST | INTEGRITY | HAPPINESS |
PEAK ATTITUDE | PASSION | PERSONAL FITNESS

THESE ARE OUR core values at GoodLife Fitness. They form our culture and are integrated into all of our member services. Our employees—or associates, as they are referred to at GoodLife—focus first and foremost on serving our members. They are interested in helping you, our members, become stronger, healthier, and happier. They have the important job of motivating and coaching you, and celebrating with you, as you achieve, maintain, or exceed your goals!

GoodLife Fitness:
A Success Story to Help You

WHEN GOODLIFE FIRST opened in 1979 in London, Ontario, it was a small fitness club measuring just 2,000 square feet. Now, in 2015, GoodLife has over 350 clubs, stretching from Newfoundland to British Columbia, more than 1.2 million members, and over 13,000 staff. One in every 34 Canadians is a GoodLife member.

GIVING TO CARDIAC REHABILITATION AND PREVENTION

IN AN INNOVATIVE collaboration—the first of its kind in Canada—GoodLife Fitness joined forces in 2012 with University Health Network, which includes Toronto General Hospital, Toronto Western Hospital, Peter Munk Cardiac Centre, and the Toronto Rehabilitation Institute. This collaboration is enabling great strides in joint private-public efforts in cardiac rehabilitation.

Why is cardiac rehab important? Cardiac rehab is a fundamental step in the recovery and management of people living with heart disease. The difference means improving survival rates by as much as 50 percent. Those who participate in rehabilitation and follow a good program of activity, nutrition, smoking cessation, and taking their medications not only have a much increased chance of survival but enjoy a much higher quality of life. One of our club managers in the Calgary area, Heather, shared this story with us:

> I remember waking up and seeing several grey-haired elderly people all around the room. Not to be rude or mean, but I felt I was in a seniors' home. I was 39 years old. A nurse came in and asked how I was

feeling. Apparently I had had two heart attacks, the second being massive. I coded twice and was brought back with the paddles on both occasions.

Still, it did not sink in until I grabbed a pillow from behind my head and tried to throw it to the chair at the foot of the bed. I felt completely drained just from the attempt. Immediately I realized my body was not the same, and I would not be able to do things like I used to.

Or so I thought.

I spent two weeks in cardiac care, and started cardiac rehabilitation after I was discharged. I felt devastated and alone, with a deep sadness for the physical and emotional person I used to be. She was gone. I was afraid to go to sleep in case I didn't wake up. I no longer had the confidence in my own body to do the simplest of everyday tasks.

The first week I got home, I tried unloading my dishwasher and had to lie down for a full day. Before I had even begun to accept the mental aspect of having had heart attacks, the physical aspect was overwhelming. Although cardiac rehab was helping me, there was the fear of what I was going to do after.

How would I cope? How would I know what I could and couldn't do? Could and couldn't eat? So many questions.

It was all just too much and too soon, but the one thing that made sense—that helped me—was only a four- to six-week program with guidance from doctors and a trained specialist. Depression, fear, and an overwhelming feeling of doom and gloom overcame me. It was extremely hard for me to see my way out of it all. Heart disease. People die from it.

A friend of mine talked me into going to a GoodLife club, and I fought it every step of the way. I was given the book *Living the Good Life* by David Patchell-Evans. At the time I felt that I had been treading water with my head barely above water and someone just threw me a lifeline. The book reached deep within, and I started to see a ray of hope.

I went back to the gym the next day, made a three-year commitment, and, with the help of several employees there, began this fantastic journey back to myself, to the girl I had lost through heart disease.

Every day I stood on that treadmill or rode an exercise bike, I had confidence to face the day and the week and pretty soon I was helping others. I was alive better than ever and not just existing and living with a pending sense of death.

As my fitness journey continued, I got a job at GoodLife and loved it. I was made for it! So much so that I tell people I am blessed to have had heart disease, as it led me to this tremendous man and company.

I had already lost one sister to heart disease and, sadly, a couple years later lost another. One died instantly from a massive heart attack. The other

suffered horribly and finally succumbed to conges-
tive heart failure.

This made me all the more determined.

I met Patch in 2010 and was thrilled in 2014 when
he invited me to share my story at the celebration of
GoodLife's partnership with the Peter Munk Cardiac
Centre (PMCC) at University Health Network
(UHN) in Toronto.

Exercise saves lives. Exercise gives you emotional
strength. No two ways about it! I am living proof.

GoodLife's donation of $5 million to the University Health
Network also established the GoodLife Fitness Centre
of Excellence in Cardiovascular Rehabilitation Medicine
along with the GoodLife Fitness Chair in Cardiovascular
Rehabilitation and Prevention.

The goal of the collaboration is to facilitate the highest
quality of research and care in cardiac rehabilitation by
funding groundbreaking research and optimal care, revital-
izing the PMCC Cardiovascular Rehabilitation Unit, and
developing a continuum of care from the acute care system
into the community. To that end, GoodLife's National
Personal Training Department worked tirelessly with UHN's
cardiology team to develop a cardiac specialization training
program. Now GoodLife's trainers will be educated by
PMCC cardiac rehabilitation experts with the goal of pro-
viding ongoing care and resources to cardiac patients under-
going cardiovascular rehabilitation and prevention.

GIVING TO KIDS: GOODLIFE KIDS FOUNDATION

GOODLIFE CARES ABOUT future generations and is making a significant investment in promoting healthy, active lifestyles among children and youth. In 1998, responding to a growing need to support and encourage fitness in children, David Patchell-Evans recruited a board of directors and launched the GoodLife Kids Foundation.

GoodLife Kids Foundation is a private charitable foundation with a vision for every Canadian kid to have the opportunity to live a fit and healthy good life. GoodLife staff, members, and corporate partners annually support the foundation through special events such as Spin4Kids Plus, a one-day fitness event hosted by GoodLife Fitness clubs across Canada. This is a fun, energetic, and volunteer-driven event where members, supporters, and staff spin, groove, and move.

For further information about programs, including support for physical activity for special needs, please visit GoodLifeKids.com.

GIVING TO AUTISM

DECEMBER 16, 2014, was an incredibly moving day for David Patchell-Evans, as he records here:

> I was standing on a plot of land located on the seawall in Richmond, BC. Given the time of year it was understandable that the area was buffeted by a cold rain and blustery winds, and the day, at 3:00 p.m., was turning to dusk. Yet the weather could not even begin to dampen the spirits of the 150 volunteers, government officials, and families standing shoulder-to-shoulder under a huge white tent lit by spotlights.
>
> The cause for celebration was the groundbreaking for the GoodLife Fitness Family Autism Hub. This new centre of excellence will bring together state-of-the-art research, information, learning, treatment, and support systems to meet the needs of families in British Columbia affected by Autism Spectrum Disorder (ASD). It will also act as a model and resource for all Canadians and people around the world.
>
> I was humbled to be a part of this day. My wife, Silken, and I spoke from our hearts about our personal and sometimes public journey with autism and then dug in with shovels in hand and helped break ground.

GIVING TO THE KILEE PATCHELL-EVANS AUTISM RESEARCH GROUP

IN 2003, a mutual friend introduced David Patchell-Evans to Dr. Derrick MacFabe, a neuroscientist based in London, Ontario. At the time, Dr. MacFabe had an as-yet-untested theory about the cause of autism, and Patch had a daughter newly diagnosed with autism. Patch was searching for answers—Dr. McCabe was searching for help to fund his research. A few hours and a handshake later, Patch had promised to fund Dr. MacFabe's research, on the condition that *the research had to be conducted openly, with as much collaboration with other scientists/researchers as possible.* The Kilee Patchell-Evans Autism Research Group was established.

Since then David Patchell-Evans has donated $5 million to support this research. Statistics for 2014, published by the CDC (Centers for Disease Control and Prevention), report Autism Spectrum Disorder now affects one in every 67 Canadians.

In 2007 Patch was awarded the Canadian Medical Association Medal of Honour—the highest honour given outside the medical profession in Canada—for his support of autism research and education. That same year, Dr.

MacFabe's research team received the Top 50 Scientific Discoveries in Canada award from NSERC (Natural Sciences and Engineering Research Council of Canada).

In 2011, David Suzuki highlighted Dr. MacFabe's work in the documentary "The Autism Enigma" on CBC's *The Nature of Things*.

By January 2013, Dr. MacFabe and Dr. Richard Frye (University of Arkansas), in a large clinical study, developed a number of valid biomarkers (blood tests) for early identification of autism, or persons at risk, which may result in early detection. It also heralded novel treatments (related to diet, metabolism, antibiotics, gut function) to treat or prevent autistic symptoms.

In 2014, Patch undertook to be a more public advocate of help for autism, writing Prime Minister Stephen Harper and all 312 Members of Parliament with a pledge of $10 million if the government would follow suit with matching funds. Patch has also been a past chair of Autism Canada and has attended meetings in Ottawa with the government and CASDA (the Canadian Autism Spectrum Disorders Alliance), representing 54 autism charities and stakeholder groups.

In 2014/2015 Dr. MacFabe will share his research at conferences on four continents.

Patch and Dr. MacFabe are united in their belief that no one group can do this alone—communities, schools, health care systems, and governments must work together. They believe Canada can become the worldwide leader in autism research, development, and treatment, building human potential in what is already the best country in the world.

To read more about this important research, visit psychology.uwo.ca/autism/

All proceeds from the sale of this book support autism.

RECOGNITION

GOODLIFE FITNESS HAS won an impressive array of awards, including:

- *Canada's 50 Best Managed Companies, Platinum Club member*
- *Canada's 10 Most Admired Corporate Cultures award, Platinum*
- *Canada's Top 10 Passion Capitalists* (for great corporate citizenry)
- *Achievers 50 Most Engaged Workplaces*™
- *Business Achievement Award*
- *Best Buddies Top Employer of the Year* (for workplace inclusion of people with intellectual disabilities)
- *Canada's Passion Capitalists Award*, National Winner, BNN, National/Financial Post
- *City of London and the London Economic Development Corporation Award* (for industry leadership, innovation, growth, and contribution to the community)
- Recognition from The Gathering in 2015 as one of the nine global cult brands with exceptional brand loyalty and customer devotion

OUR FOUNDER AND CEO, Dr. David Patchell-Evans—or Patch, as he prefers to be called—has also achieved many honours, including:

- Honorary Doctorate, Western University
- *Most Innovative CEO of the Year Canada*, Canadian Business Magazine
- *Medal of Honour*, Canadian Medical Association, for support of autism research
- International Entrepreneur of the Year Institute special citation for Customer Driven Focus
- *Icon Business Achievement Award* from the London Chamber of Commerce
- Western University *Alumni Award of Merit*
- Induction into the Junior Achievement Business Hall of Fame
- *CVCA Entrepreneur of the Year Award*
- *Upper Canada Medal*, awarded by University Health Network (UHN) for contributions in support of the public good
- *Icon Business Achievement Award* from the London Chamber of Commerce

THE GREAT THINGS GOODLIFE HAS TO OFFER YOU

UNBELIEVABLE OPPORTUNITIES AND experiences await you at GoodLife Fitness: many different forms of strength training and many different types of fitness classes and cardiovascular training. So the key is to keep it simple. Just say to yourself, "Look, all I really need to do is some strength and some cardio, and I don't need to spend a lot of time—only 20 to 30 minutes three times a week." You don't need to change your entire schedule—just a little change will make your life a whole lot better.

Whether you are just getting started on fitness, challenging yourself to new levels, or focused on improving your health and well-being, we welcome you! To learn about all the programs GoodLife has to offer, including exclusive Group Exercise programs, Team Training, Personal Training, Corporate Wellness, Massage, and Chiropractic, or our exclusive Lifechanger program, visit us in person at any club or visit the website below.

If you are looking for a great career in our fitness clubs, health centres, or home office, and if you live to help people achieve their goals, please visit **goodlifefitness.com**.